THE BIT'
OF TI

CW01431475

GIULIA CAMINITO

translated by

HOPE CAMPBELL GUSTAFSON

In the 1990s, Gaia's family moves from the neglected peripheries of Rome to an idyllic lakeside town in search of a new life that will lift them out of poverty. Each of them bears their own scars: Gaia's mother is fiercely determined to secure a better future for her children at any cost; her father, a once proud man, now suffers in bitter silence after a devastating accident; and her young twin brothers wordlessly bear witness to a family in decay.

When Gaia meets two local girls, Agata and Carlotta, the trio builds a fragile friendship. Gaia's encounters with callous boys and contemptuous teachers convince her that she might always be an outsider—excluded from a privileged life and beyond the possibility of happiness.

Winner of the Campiello Prize, *The Bitter Water of the Lake* is an unflinching portrait of a generation striving to make a place for themselves in a world markedly different from the one their parents promised them.

'It is impossible not to be swept away by this novel of extraordinary elegance and maturity, not to keep thinking about its many hearts.'

'A luminous and powerful voice . . . a voice so unique that we haven't heard anything like it in a long time. You can't miss it.'

'A sharpness in style that aptly conveys the challenges of growing up—acknowledging true friends over fair-weather ones and finding pride in one's authentic self.'

'If the torments of adolescence are universal, the harsh poetry of *The Bitter Water of the Lake* gracefully reminds us how it is a unique drama for each individual.'

'*The Bitter Water of the Lake* is an intense story, elegant and precise.'

'Giulia Caminito constructs characters the readers feel invested in, characters who show their deepest scars.'

'In this visionary and original novel, so lyrical and lush in its prose, the protagonist Gaia endures tragedies, separations, and a ferocious destiny that seems to deny any possibility of redemption.'

THE INDIGO PRESS
50 Albemarle Street
London W1S 4BD
www.theindigopress.com

The Indigo Press Publishing Limited Reg. No. 10995574
Registered Office: Wellesley House, Duke of Wellington Avenue,
Royal Arsenal, London SE18 6SS

First published in Great Britain in 2025 by The Indigo Press

Originally published in Italian under the title *L'acqua del lago non è mai dolce*
© 2021 Giunti Editore S.p.A. / Bompiani. Published by special arrangement
with Giulia Caminito in conjunction with her duly appointed agent
MalaTesta Literary Agency and the co-agent 2 Seas Literary Agency

First published in English in the USA by Spiegel and Grau in 2025

A CIP catalogue record for this book is available from the British Library

ISBN: 978-1917378260
eBook ISBN: 978-1917378277

Cover design © Sarah Schulte
Apartment – istock © Grand Warszawski
Woman – istock © Wirestock
Star sticker – istock © kyoshino
Rose from the book *Everybody's Flower Garden* by Harry Higgott Thomas
Art direction by House of Thought
Offset by Tetragon, London
Printed and bound in Great Britain by Clays Ltd, Elcograf S.p.A.

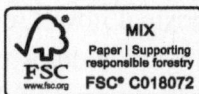

FSC
www.fsc.org
MIX
Paper | Supporting
responsible forestry
FSC® C018072

EU GPSR authorised representative
Logos Europe, 9 rue Nicolas Poussin, 17000, La Rochelle, France
e-mail: contact@logoseurope.eu

1 3 5 7 9 8 6 4 2

THE BITTER WATER OF THE LAKE

GIULIA CAMINITO

translated by

HOPE CAMPBELL GUSTAFSON

THE
INDIGO
PRESS

All lives begin with a woman, as did mine—a woman with red hair who enters a room wearing a linen suit pulled out of her closet for the occasion. She'd bought it at the stall in Porta Portese, the good one with the discounted designer clothes—not the clothes that all cost very little, but those with the sign that says: PRICES VARY.

The woman is my mother and she's clutching a black leather briefcase in her left hand. She styled her hair herself with curlers and hair spray, did her bangs with a brush. She has green-and-yellow eyes and confirmation-style shoes on her feet. She walks in and the room feels small.

Clerks are sitting at their desks. My mother spent three hours waiting outside on the corner, the briefcase held against her chest, and when she tells it she says her legs were butter and her spit sour.

She approaches, swaying her hips. The perfume she put on to mask the smell of the lentils she made for lunch arrives before she does, and she says: I'm here to see Dottoressa Ragni, I have an appointment.

She'd repeated that phrase to herself in the mirror and on the tram and in the elevator and on the corner: I have an appointment. In a sweet tone, a cheerful tone, a firm tone, in a whisper, as if it were completely normal, and now she says it to a young woman with no wedding ring and hair tied back, who observes her and sees how her linen suit is a bit crumpled and the leather briefcase is worn away at the handle.

The young woman looks down at the appointment book on the desk in front of her: May I ask your name?

Antonia Colombo, my mother says.

The young woman carefully checks Dottoressa Ragni's schedule, scans the page with her finger and searches for Colombo, but can't find it.

Your name isn't here, ma'am.

My mother sneers. It's something she had carefully thought through. She'd wondered what face to make in that exact moment— she'd had to consider every instant, to visualize what was going to happen in detail. Sneering comes easily to her, as if she were a busy woman, bothered by other people's incompetence, by delays.

My mother says: Look, miss, I made my appointment over a week ago, I'm a lawyer and Dottoressa Ragni assured me she'd be in today, we're behind with the delivery of the deeds.

My mother's sneer is crooked and her impatience is real, as real as shoes that are too tight or tall, sweaty men on the tram.

The two exchange more words and Antonia Colombo insists, certain it's the right thing to do: take up space and never move again.

The young woman is persuaded. This red-haired woman seems sure of what she says and no one in the office has so much as looked up from the papers in front of them, since an argument hasn't broken out yet. So the young woman opens the door with the DOTTORESSA RAGNI plaque for my mother, who walks right through—the threshold to her future.

She sees a third woman, dressed in a skirt-and-blazer set with green polka dots on a black background, and waits for the door to close behind her.

She and the dottoressa study each other. The latter has her hands in a drawer she quickly closes. Behind her is a bookcase packed with legal volumes, and my mother knows she will never in her life be able to have that much paper, because paper takes up space and costs money.

Sorry, who are you? asks Dottoressa Ragni, crossing her legs.

Antonia Colombo, my mother responds and adds: We do not know each other and I do not have an appointment.

A heavy silence fills the air for several seconds until Antonia speaks again.

You don't know me but you have my housing-request paperwork on your desk, I'm certain it's there, in that pile—I'm in there too. I live on Via Monterotto 63, or actually, I don't live there because my residence isn't recognized, and we're in a twenty-square-meter basement, the bills aren't in my name, and I pay a fine for being a tenant. I paid in advance to stay there and I want to be brought into compliance. It's already been five years.

The dottoressa gets up from her chair, revealing that she's not very tall. She takes her glasses off—they're round and tortoiseshell—and angrily tosses them onto her desk, yelling at my mother to get out.

My mother says: I've gone to your offices, all of them, I've brought the documents you asked for, I married the man who lived with me, I had him adopt my son, I got pregnant, I started a family, and I meet all the requirements.

The dottoressa begins punching numbers on her phone, then throws the receiver down, threatens to call the police, and tells my mother she must leave immediately. How dare you come in here under false pretenses? She says it louder: How dare you?

Then my mother sits down on the ground and crosses her legs. Her linen skirt rides up her white, freckle-covered thighs, she raises her hands above her head and says: I am here. I'm here for my house.

And she does not move, her arms are rigid, her hands open wide. The briefcase is on the ground and it's empty. My mother is not a lawyer and she doesn't have appointments with people who matter. She has a house that she's cleared of mice and cockroaches and syringes and she wants a solution.

The dottoressa moves away from her desk and past my mother, purposely bumping into her with a knee before opening the door, and she calls for help in the office, saying: There's a crazy lady sitting on the floor, get her out of here.

The young woman from earlier and the doorman and the janitor and some other men rush in and find this tree trunk of a woman— my mother—with her hands raised toward the ceiling and her linen skirt riding up all the way. She has a face like marble and she's screaming insults at the top of her lungs.

She doesn't think they know what it means to reach the point when you can no longer take it, after one two three four five ten social workers, one two three four five ten post offices, one two three four five ten public attorneys, one two three four five ten public housing employees, one two three four five ten forms to fill out, one two three four five ten fines and bills and reprimands and threats.

They raise her up and move her, lifting her by her arms and legs. Her blouse opens and reveals a bra without underwire, swollen breasts. Her skirt rips and her underwear peeks out. My mother has already torn her good suit to shreds and she kicks and screams, like a wild beast.

It's as if I were there, standing, watching her from the corner of the room. I judge her and I do not forgive her.

1

Home Is Where the Heart Is

We live in a neighborhood that my mother doesn't like calling the outskirts, since to be on the outskirts you have to know what your center is, but we never see that center. I have never visited the Colosseum, the Sistine Chapel, the Vatican, Villa Borghese, Piazza del Popolo. We don't go on school trips, and when I do go out, it's with my mother to our neighborhood market.

What I cherish most about our house—five meters wide and four meters long—is the concrete courtyard and the flower beds, where there's only grass. No one ever thought to put flowers in them, and even my mother refused to, because planting means staying.

Our house is a kitchen in a closet, it's a cot that pulls out from under Mariano's bed, it's an electric radiator to be turned on low (and only when it's truly cold), it's a poster of the Beatles above the table where we eat and our four chairs. It's hearing my parents' bed squeak when they're doing you-know-what because there's just one room and it's not like you can go outside or shut yourself in the bathroom. Even from the bathroom and from outside, you can hear everything.

The house is me as a girl, and that concrete courtyard is all I know. I inhabit it like a palace with my brother. It's ours and no one else's— we dig, jump, cook plants and ants, and on the ground we trace numbers and lines and triangles and squares with pieces of chalk from school. We sit in them and say they are ours. We live there, inside the symbols on the ground that we drew.

H-O-M-E, we say, and all it takes is a few lines to make the walls and the roof, the windows, the door.

That place, the land of our games and earliest fantasies, only exists because of our mother. Before her, it was home to cockroaches, a few mice, and syringes tossed through the fence from the street or left behind by someone sleeping in the doorway.

Our mother pulled on tall rubber boots—borrowed from my father—to pick them up one by one and burn them before throwing them out. If you find a syringe, my mother always says, you have to get rid of it because if a child were to fall on it, it'd be partially your fault—you ignored it.

She got some poison, had my father bring a shovel home from the construction site, and set about hunting, killing, eradicating the pests. After months of work, the courtyard onto which the toothless mouth of our basement apartment opens has been reclaimed and she takes us by the hand and leads us there, saying: Play.

To get that house, my mother had asked her grandma for some money to buy out the relatives of an old lady who had died there. In a working-class neighborhood of heroin addicts and dying old people, no one would have ever bought that moldy dump and my mother never would've had the money to buy it anyway, so she came to an agreement with the owners and began getting all her paperwork in order to find another place and establish legal residence there, at least temporarily.

She'd thought it wouldn't take too long, that somehow she'd be able to make it happen, that they would find us a new house while we stayed there and waited.

So we wait. We wait so long that eventually my mother gives in and starts scrubbing and fixing the floor and painting the ceiling and making it so the water drains better in the tub—all because the municipality of Rome doesn't want to give us a home.

Everything balances on something that is ready to collapse yet clings with its very last root to the crumbly soil, until my mother gets pregnant again and my father, who is not Mariano's father, is injured at work: he falls from a scaffold and is paralyzed.

Disability documents are added to the marriage and adoption papers. Alongside claims for unemployment benefits, there are those for a large family and others for sending my little brothers to day care. We live by asking the city, the mayor, Italy, to help us and shelter us and protect us and not forget us. Our lives are a perpetual prayer.

I'm six when the twins are born, and Mariano hates us all, especially the father who is not his and who has been transformed from a gruff man into a bulky and tiring accessory—an oven that no longer works, a vacuum that collects nothing off the floor, a hot-water heater that leaves you to shower in the cold after only five minutes. He's a piece of junk and Mariano wants to throw him away.

My father, once known for his savage blows and his high sex drive, is now stuck in a wheelchair, which my mother got from some relatives at the hospital. He lifts his legs up one at a time and no longer eats his dinner. What's the point of eating anyway.

In our house there is a stationary man who is like a statue, like marble, floor tiles, a doorframe, or the low walls bordering the building; there is also a busy woman who picks things up, who moves things around, polishes, repairs, glues, poisons, pushes water outside with a broom when heavy rains flood the house. The stationary man is my father, and the other person, the tireless one, is the red-haired woman whose name is Antonia Colombo.

I don't have toys and I have few friends. I'm given everything's cheap imitation: a doll sewn from fabric scraps, a folder covered in another girl's doodles, shoes brought home from the market in a plastic bag—without a box and with their soles already worn—mandarin oranges instead of Christmas lights, and instead of Barbies, images of them cut out of magazines.

I feel like we're scrap material, useless cards in a complicated game, chipped marbles that no longer roll—we're left motionless on the ground, like my father, who fell from inadequate scaffolding at an illegal construction site, without a contract and without insurance. From down below, from where we have plummeted, we can see the others putting gemstone necklaces around their necks.

The twins are tiny, noisy creatures that sleep in an enormous box full of blankets set on top of the kitchen table, and the smell of their diapers blends with that of the soup.

Mariano and I don't understand why we're still there, why we've never tried to escape. We plan it out in secret, me and my dark-haired brother—the moment we'll run away—and yet we're never quite ready to duck out, to turn the corner of our lives.

We're the kind of people who barely know the geography of Lazio—
our region—or the streets of Rome—our city—because the boundaries of our movements are confined to our neighborhood. Beyond
it, things cost too much for us, and no one outside of our neighborhood would extend credit to my mother or exchange bread and prosciutto for a day's labor.

My mother's theory: If they don't know you, they won't help you.
So we stay where people know who we are, where she can weave
small and large webs of safety and familiarity.

Mariano is the oldest, and he experienced each of us as an intru-
sion between him and Antonia, who for a while was a single mother.
The two of them had lived as one body in order to survive.

My brother tolerates me because I'm not a crybaby and because
I listen to him. I let him unload fairy tales and demons on me, dark
and terrible stories, and adventures in which the girl always dies and
the wolf always wins. There are four years between us, which feel like
many more when you're young. Those four years make him seem like
an adult to me, almost ancient. He's the one who steps in whenever
anyone bothers me. I can't stand the other girls at school and look at
them with disdain. They all seem to have something I lack, but I still
haven't figured out my own way to fight them.

There's a blonde girl—I think she's Austrian—who calls me Bat
Beak because, as she puts it, I have protruding lips. So I stand on my
tiptoes in the bathroom at home to check. It really doesn't seem to
me like I have any deformities, and I know that bats were once mice
and not ducks, but children's insults don't have to make sense to hurt.
Being different—defective—harms you; staying perfectly in line

helps you blend in and avoid notice. Some of us are ruined enough as it is. We can't afford to have beaks or conspicuous ears.

When I tell Mariano about it, he shows up outside my school, asks me to point out which girl it is, and yells at her: Keep your mouth shut, moron. Then he punches her.

I feel a rush of admiration for him. He silenced her cruelty with one gesture. I tuck his short temper away in my treasure chest.

The incident isn't appreciated by my teachers or my mother, who ties Mariano's hands behind his back for a couple of days, telling him he has to do without them and ask us for help with the tasks he can't do on his own. If he isn't able to use his hands properly, then he won't use them at all.

Antonia finds unorthodox solutions to problems. She rarely hits or kicks us—instead, she prefers taking something away from us. If we yell in the house, she won't make dinner; if we choose to play our games instead of helping her with the twins, she won't pack us a snack for school or she confiscates our pencil cases. She goes on strikes and resists in other ways.

Who knows where she got her ideas, maybe from my grandma, maybe from life, or maybe they were her own. She has no religion, she's lost her political party, she's only certain about justice. She has a strong fixation on things that are just.

I am fascinated by flowers, not the few that spontaneously sprout in our courtyard—those fragile little springtime daisies—but the roses in other people's gardens, the jasmine, the hydrangeas, the flowers I see peeking out while passing by on the sidewalk behind my mother, flowers I want to pick.

Then one day I go for it, because I want to steep the petals of those roses in a plastic bottle filled with water, like my classmates do, before they show off their smelly but precious homemade perfumes at school. Antonia sees me pick a rose that was sticking through a fence and we start arguing.

You cannot take what isn't yours, she scolds.

But it was on the street and the street is everyone's, I reply.

That makes you even more of a thief, my mother snarls. What belongs to everyone is not to be touched.

Breaking or damaging things is a sacrilege, one my mother always seeks to remedy immediately by finding ways to repair or reuse whatever has been broken. But when it comes to what belongs to everyone, she is uncompromising: Do not walk on the grass in the park, do not litter, do not pick roses from gardens, do not ruin library books.

Books are her greatest obsession, because at home, where we don't have a television—only a radio—the only pastime is reading, especially ever since my father has either been in bed or in his chair. And because we don't have the space or money for books, we read books that belong to everyone and treat them like relics—they're kept neatly stacked, my mother writes down all their due dates and badgers us to finish and return them on time. She checks to make sure we haven't stained or creased them, and if we have, she drags us to the library to apologize to the librarian and the other children and then she pays for them. Even if they tell her it's not necessary, she replies: Of course it's necessary.

When I dare to point out that it seems like the things that belong to everyone actually belong to no one, she tells me: Get that idea out of your head right now or you'll grow up to be a very bad woman.

Antonia no longer dresses up. She goes there in the same clothes she wears at home, all sweaty with her hair in a clip. Her face is round and her temples are narrow. Her eyes have long lashes and her nose doesn't stand out but it doesn't blend in either. She isn't skinny, and she's not overweight. She has a healthy body.

She always says that what's important is to look healthy: Chicken legs aren't good, sunken faces are scary.

Antonia decided that to get what she wants, she has to insist. She stepped onto the stage like a spotlight that detaches from the ceiling and crashes onto the set: unwanted and dangerous. She was supposed to shine a light on others but now is trying to steal the show.

She is a dysfunctional, desperate, and disaffected woman, and she's carrying a bundle of documents. She identified a clerk who seems friendlier than the rest and wrote his name down on a slip of paper, last name first: Murri Franco.

Now listen to me, Murri Franco, I am Colombo Antonia, and until you help me, I'll keep coming back here and asking for you, my mother declares, handing him her folders, one after the other.

Murri Franco tries to be polite: You know, ma'am, you've come in here before under false pretenses and our manager hasn't forgotten you. It's unlikely that this will end in your favor.

Colombo Antonia does not give in: Then we'll put my paperwork on that desk fifty times over until I've become so inconvenient that I can no longer be ignored. I have four children and a disabled husband at home.

For the next one two three months, she knows that if she goes to a new clerk, she'll have to start all over again. If she doesn't see Murri Franco at his desk, she tells them she'll be back the next day or she makes another appointment.

And when she comes home, she talks about Franco as if he were the pharmacist or a newspaper vendor—a familiar man from a known and reassuring world. We have no idea what he looks like. He feels like an intruder. We don't understand what he's doing for our mother, and we start to get jealous, Mariano especially.

Your dad never says anything about her seeing that guy all the time, my brother says to me one day, as if it were my fault for having a father when he doesn't or, at least, one that he doesn't want.

What's he supposed to say? I respond and look over at my father. He's sitting, the wheels of his chair are beached against a leg of the table and he has *il manifesto* open across his knees. He's been stuck on the same page for at least half an hour and I wonder if he's forgotten what he's reading.

Something, Mariano replies and casts disapproving eyes on him, the same look he always gives him.

Papà is burned-out, he's spent. I go over to him and place a hand on his knee even though he can't feel it, and I ask who this Franco guy is and if there's anything he wants to say to him.

Papà doesn't look at me but he says: Tell your brother to shut up.

He and Mariano face off—the former from his chair, the latter from his bed—because they're always in the same room, they can't escape, they can't pretend they didn't hear what the other said.

They arrested her, my father adds, while Mariano angrily pulls on his sneakers. He's going on a run.

Who? I ask, looking down at the newspaper.

That woman, the manager, my father explains, but I don't know what a manager is or what they manage, so I search the printed words for a clue and I read the name under his finger: Vittoria Ragni.

I don't know who she is. I read that name over and over—Vittoria Ragni—I even say it out loud when my mother walks in: Vittoria Ragni. She's carrying a jug of floor cleaner. She never comes home empty-handed. She brings us glass jars, plastic bottles, pieces of plywood, things other people no longer need but we definitely do.

Vittoria Ragni, what? she asks, setting the jug down on the table where we are. Mariano, where are you going? she says, but Mariano ignores her and heads outside, which means he's not there to witness our mother's first great satisfaction. He doesn't see her face when her forehead wrinkles relax. He can't appreciate the gleam in her eyes, her lips curling at the corners.

Antonia rips the newspaper out of my father's hands and reads, rereads, then I see tremors sprouting from her smile. I see my mother cry.

I stare at her, stunned. I've hardly ever seen her cry—not in the hospital while giving birth to the twins, not even when her grandma died, or when my father fell.

She's under investigation. They're sending her to prison, she says through her tears, and I can't tell whether she's happy or sad.

Was she a friend of yours? I ask shyly, and she bursts into laughter. Her eyes are still wet but she's laughing hard.

Antonia has to show them what we're missing. She shows them how the hot water never comes, the outlets have exposed electrical wires, there's a lack of space to move around in, and the natural light barely enters. And yet while those people are there she keeps repeating: We're getting by, at least it's all clean.

The new manager is a woman with a background in social work, and when she reads in our file that there are four children living in twenty square meters, she takes a red pen and on the first page writes: URGENT.

They take on our case and come inspect where we're living. They find my father sitting on the bed—he doesn't even say buongiorno—and the twins clinging to my mother's skirt, almost pulling it down. At the foot of the closet is the bag with their clothes. They sleep in a box, glued to each other. They still haven't experienced being apart.

Mariano is out in the courtyard and we hear him scream. He's pretending to be in danger. He says help help in his grown-up voice and my mother tells them: Don't worry, he just wants attention, he's fine.

There are two intruders and they make our house feel even smaller. Now it looks like a storage space or a back room, like a detergent-and-broom closet.

The police are here, Mariano yells from outside, and then he throws a firecracker on the ground.

The intruders are taking notes, they ask my mother questions about the state of the property, and when they leave, my father lies back on his side with difficulty and starts to snore. I eat a raw carrot and my mother looks out at Mariano from the doorway: You brat, she yells at him, those people work for the city! You're getting stale bread for dinner.

Two weeks later the new manager calls my mother. The waiting list for housing is long, as we know, and our paperwork has been sitting there for a while, but she wants us to leave that place, it's much too small. She found us a house, one she can't officially allocate to us but that she could give us custody of. With a signed document from her, we can live there until further notice.

My mother photocopies that piece of paper dozens of times and brings it with her to every relevant office, to the post office, the bank, the revenue agency. She keeps a copy in her wallet and one pinned to the wall. She safeguards one next to our ID cards and the little boxes with our baby teeth.

Distressed and dismayed, Mariano and I say goodbye to our square of concrete.

Our new home is in a neighborhood for people who have money. We're on Corso Trieste near all the offices and banks. We can walk to parks like Villa Torlonia and Villa Ada. It takes ten minutes to get to the famous Piper Club, and the next neighborhood over is Parioli—the richest in the entire city. In our building, which has two internal courtyards and six floors, the city only owns one apartment, the one now in our custody.

We move into the apartment with our boxes, our odds and ends, the yogurt containers we use as cactus pots, the glass bean jars that are our toothbrush holders, our clothes hangers made out of cardboard and tape, and our underwear, bunched up at the bottom of trash bags.

It has three bedrooms, a kitchen, a living area. There's a real entryway with real stairs, a real door, a real bathtub, real burners, and real shutters.

Mariano and I set two plastic bags with our wonky toys down in the middle of our room. It feels too big for us, it's almost scary.

I've slept badly ever since we moved there. I force my brother to keep the light on, and I always wake up at midnight, right on the dot, to find myself plagued by a nightmare that I can never really remember. All I know is that I usually fall and no one's there to catch me.

At night I no longer hear my father's loud breathing or the twins crying. I only see Mariano getting up and going over to the window to look down at the street below.

The upstairs neighbors start complaining about how the twins never sleep, how Mariano and I walk too quickly, how my mother turns the radio up too loud when she washes the dishes, how my father curses every morning—instead of saying, What a beautiful day, he summons all the saints down to Earth.

In the new building there's a condo association, the people who run it, and meetings we aren't allowed to attend because the house isn't really ours—we didn't buy it. Still nothing belongs to us.

The courtyard is full of roses—yellow, red, salmon colored—and fruit-bearing plants, but we can't touch them, no one can. A gardener comes every Wednesday and sprays them with something that stinks.

The first afternoon that Mariano and I play outside in the courtyard, a bucketful of water rains down on us from above. Some lady doesn't appreciate the racket we're making.

Mariano yells at her: You bitch!

And she says she's calling the police.

My mother scolds us and tells Mariano not to yell. Those people were here before us and we can't continue to act like we did in the old house. We have to adapt to other people's lives, be respectful.

Grocery shopping in the neighborhood is hard for us—it all costs too much. We started school in the middle of the year and, according to our teachers, we're so far behind that we'll have to repeat a year. They're always kicking my brother out of the classroom, and I barely speak. I respond in incomplete sentences, my handwriting is shaky, and I'm envious of all the other girls' *o*'s and *m*'s.

The only friend my mother has in our building is the doorperson, a woman from Sicily who's short and not very chatty but quick and thorough with her cleaning. She listens to everyone's complaints— their affairs, their troubles—and never shares her own. She keeps the incoming mail in order and has a board where she hangs the keys to all the apartments and cellars and to every lock in the building. They aren't labeled. Only she knows which key opens what; it's her secret.

The doorwoman's name is Nunzia and she has a daughter, Roberta, who is in a wheelchair like my father, though she didn't fall. She was born that way and can't speak well and often her head droops and her gaze turns vacant as if she were no longer there.

On the way home from school I always stop in the courtyard and, if no one is watching, I toss my backpack to the ground and go to the fountain in the center. It's white and dirty, but in the water six goldfish swim around in circles. I spend many hours with my hand submerged, trying to pet them. They slip away and then come closer, and I stir and stir the water. With my cupped hands I collect the twigs floating on the surface.

It seems like a game that shouldn't bother anyone. The fish and I make no noise, and I keep them company. I don't spill too much water, and I never drink it.

There's a spot in the garden that the sun reaches even in winter, a corner from which, if you look up, you'll see a little slice of sky— the perfect triangle to make you forget you're in the middle of the city—and that's where Nunzia situates her daughter, Roberta, in her wheelchair, because she likes the light. Their apartment, next to the concierge's station, is the smallest in the building. It doesn't have many stairs, thankfully, but it also doesn't get much air.

Roberta is a quiet girl. Sometimes she gurgles, licks her lips, elongates words, and asks questions only her mother can understand, but it takes no effort at all for her to make it clear that she wants to sit out there in the sun.

I see how many people in the building pass by without greeting her. They also glance over at me and just keep walking. They don't care about the fish. So I say: Ciao. I say it loudly, to everyone, to see what they do, whether they respond. Some mutter a buongiorno or buonasera. Others say absolutely nothing; they don't even bother responding.

There's a German woman who sternly scrutinizes us from her window, and when she comes down into the courtyard, she paces back and forth. She smiles at the other women, but not at us. Instead she looks at me, puts her hands on her hips, walks away, goes to the doorwoman, complains, and returns. One day, red in the face, she pounces on me and rips my hands from the water—she's the army, I'm a bandit.

Stop, you're ruining it, she screams. She has pale-blue eyes and a wide forehead.

All that movement scares the fish, spinning around in their cauldron, their tails rigid, their eyes desperate. Roberta squirms and stomps her feet, the German lady grips my wrist and pushes me toward the stairwell entrance, the one leading to my house.

Now go, she orders hotly, and I climb the stairs two by two and look for my mother. I find her with one twin around her neck and the other pantless, standing on the table. He's moving his bottom around so much it looks like he's dancing.

Ma', I say, all sweaty from running up the stairs. The German woman yelled at me about the fountain, she says I'm ruining it.

I've told you over and over you can't play in the courtyard. It's not like our old house. The fountain is there for decoration, you understand? It's not for play, it's to make the building look pretty, like a bow.

I was just minding my own business and watching the fish, I say. What are these stupid people doing with a pretty place no one can even touch?

And what are they doing with all their necklaces and their lace? Nothing—people aren't doing anything with anything, they make themselves pretty and that's it.

Over the next few days, I walk past the fountain, gazing over at it like a long-lost lover. The fish are jewels and the roses are rouge and no one cares about them. I quickly realize that Roberta isn't in her spot. Even though the days have been sunny, she hasn't been back in the garden. My mother notices, too, and so she goes and asks why.

She finds out it was because of the German lady. She'd told the doorwoman that her drooling daughter wasn't nice to look at, and since those people are already here—me and my family—no one would want to buy an apartment in the building ever again. We were depreciating the property value.

So my mother waits for her. She brings the twins, Mariano, and me downstairs, then she orders us to take off our shirts and stand up against the wall. She takes hers off, too. In her bra, she leans against the wall like someone sentenced to a firing squad. When the German lady arrives with her husband, my mother tells her: Until you let the girl sit in the garden again, we'll stand here every day, me and my children, without our clothes, in protest.

She yells it and people look out their windows into the courtyard. The German lady stands there immobile, like stockfish, like a coatrack, then says: I'm calling the police.

Go ahead, we're not moving. How can you deny a girl from sitting in the sun? A girl who can't walk. That's what I'll tell the police, and if they send us away we'll be back. You don't know how stubborn I can be when I want to, you really don't.

The German lady's husband intervenes while the two women are screaming at each other and we're standing there half naked, glued to the wall, Mariano in his underwear, me with my skirt lifted. We're ready for the revolution.

You see those gates? asks the German lady's husband, who's definitely at least ten years older than she is. We put them back up after the war because the Fascists had stolen them. This building has a history, he points out calmly and bitterly, and his poisonous calm seems to make my mother even angrier.

And who are the Fascists now, huh? You care about gates but not about children. You don't let them play, you don't say hi to them or give them hugs, you don't even let them sit in a corner. What kind of people are you? I nearly got AIDS just to make sure my children could play. The red-haired woman hits her chest proudly then makes a gesture of shooting up with a syringe.

The neighbors don't know what to say. They're speechless.

At the agreed-upon signal, we put our clothes back on and follow Antonia home single file. She declares that we'll be back.

And we do go back—every afternoon after school—to make a scene in the courtyard until Roberta takes up her rightful place in her patch of sun once again.

You have to insist and insist until you achieve, my mother explains to Mariano. If you insist, you'll get what you want. She watches Roberta in her terry bib, waving her hands in the air and turning her wrists. She looks happy.

Our mother is like the hero in a comic strip, like Anna Magnani in the movies. She's someone who makes noise, who never surrenders, who forces everyone else to hold their tongues.

Mariano and I are there in the hallway with short trousers and stiff calves, staring our fear straight in the eye: the fear that we will not end up like Antonia, that we will never be enough, that we will never win a single battle.

2

The Sunken Nativity Scene

One morning I walk into the kitchen and Antonia hands me a pea-green hat with a lopsided brim and says: I'm taking you somewhere.

Where's Mariano? I ask, because his breakfast mug isn't on the table.

Out, he's not coming, my mother responds bluntly. Get dressed, it's late.

And the twins and Papà? I ask.

The doorwoman will keep an eye on them. You have freckles on your nose, she adds, inspecting my face as though seeing it for the first time.

I am the small her and she is the big me: same frizzy red hair, same mud-green eyes, same inability to color coordinate, same way of not knowing how to drink from narrow glasses, and freckles on our noses. Each of our shared characteristics is a mortal defect. Our freckles are worse than pimples, our eyes are neither truly green nor properly brown, our pale skin invites illness, and our hair—the worst trait of them all—leads to disaster.

My mother and I take the bus and two metros as far as Valle Aurelia, then from there a regional train on a recently renovated line. It feels like we're embarking on a galactic journey. My pink terry shorts are a space suit and my lopsided hat is the helmet through which I can see the stars.

The seats have a small diamond pattern on them and the electric-blue headrests have a bulge on one side so that if you lean your temple against it you can take a nap.

There's a little metal container you can use to throw out papers or trash. It makes a sharp sound when you close it and reminds me of a mechanical shark's mouth. I play with it, opening and closing it, going *tac tac*, until a woman nearby snorts and my mother threatens me, saying she'll take my hat away and then I'll get too much sun.

The air-conditioning comes up from below and our feet get cold inside our canvas shoes. The stations have plexiglass windows and green framework. When I ask where we are so I can understand just how far from home we're going, Antonia says: On the train, and ends the conversation there.

She brought crossword puzzles with her and fills them out without asking for my help. I peek. She just wrote the word *constellation* vertically.

Which?

Which what?

Which constellation?

I don't know the stars.

Could be the Big Dipper.

She doesn't respond. She's already onto the next word, twenty-seven across.

I can't remember ever traveling like this except to go see Grandma in Ostia, something we rarely do because it means my father is home alone. Also my grandma can't stand the twins, and my mother thinks Mariano will end up getting stabbed by a syringe when he walks by the beach clubs at night.

Where are we going? I ask Antonia while rubbing my thighs back and forth against the padded, rough seats.

To see a house, she responds as if she were talking about a beach umbrella or chair, about something common.

Whose house? I ask.

Our house, Antonia replies, and I feel like she's pranking me. Her red hair is lying, and the train is going to leave us stranded in the desert.

We don't have houses that belong to us, only houses that someone else lets us live in as a courtesy. I say courtesy so that I don't say charity, but maybe charity is the right word, or maybe not—maybe it's assistance, or support, or necessity. Maybe the word is lie.

With my eyes wide-open I read the names of all the stops aloud and Antonia tells me that we're north of Rome. That's Via Cassia and this is the Cesano station, near the military barracks. It feels like we're crossing an entire continent. We'll encounter different peoples and nations, we'll invade enemy territories.

The next station's blue sign says ANGUILLARA SABAZIA and my mother forces me to get off the train. I feel my feet resisting, but I keep quiet. The train departs, and we ask for directions.

How far is it to the lake? Antonia asks, and we find out that it's four kilometers away and there are no buses; either we go by foot or we ask for a ride.

I follow my mother out of the station. In front of us are shelters for when it rains, a newsstand, a kiosk for espressos and cappuccinos, the intersection of two small streets, and the countryside opening up on either side.

Farther ahead there's a church. It's ugly and sad. You can tell it was built recently. It's shaped like a circus tent and has openwork walls and a glass door with the kind of handles a hospital would have—only the cross on the roof reveals its function. Behind it are the parish sports fields and, in front, a piazza with an already-broken fountain.

Antonia stands there and waits for someone to stop and offer us a ride. She makes stiff gestures, doesn't smile, and no one even looks our way. She squeezes my hand as she would a gun.

My mother hardly ever has low-cut or tight-fitting clothes; she wears knee-length shorts with pockets at the thighs and men's crew-neck T-shirts with construction-company logos and phone numbers on them. My father says she looks like she works for one.

The construction worker in question and I have red hair and we're standing still like people who need to pray and wait for an answer. Three cars in total pass us on the street, no one stops.

I tell Antonia: Let's go home now.

She gets upset and pulls me in close, saying with conviction: Don't be silly, this place is beautiful. There's the lake.

From the outside, the building looks like a small-scale factory, like it could produce cans of tuna or shoes with thick laces, like it has dumpsters in the back and workers who clock in every morning at seven, but it's really just a public housing complex. Nearby there are stand-alone houses, two small parks for babies and dogs, and a rectangular piazzale paved with concrete that gleams like Hawaii sand.

It faces the town's main road, where there's a building-supply store, an optician offering two-for-one deals, and a house under construction.

The windows are all at the same height. The square balconies can fit, at most, a small table and two stools, an aloe plant and a broom stand, and the front door leads to symmetrical stairwells—it's a compact building, neither old nor new, like a middle-aged woman who doesn't dress in ruffles and pearls yet still prefers to cover the dark circles under her eyes before going out in public.

Antonia leads me up to the third floor, and a woman in a floral dress—the kind that crosses in the front with a V-neck but ties in the back like an apron—shakes our hands and smiles. She smiles widely, with the kind of sinister enthusiasm that suggests a robbery is about to happen.

My mother introduces her to me and the woman says: It's a pleasure. Mirella.

I just say my name without *It's a pleasure*.

This apartment is almost as big as the one on Corso Trieste, she's keen to stress, and it has a functional little balcony, fantastic for the summer, convenient for hanging your clothes out to dry. The kitchen is furnished and the gas stove is up to code, the lady says. It's a calm place, she continues, public housing here isn't like public housing in Rome; here families actually work, children play in the park. The bathroom, according to her, is spacious and there's a tub so my father can, with only a few adjustments, wash himself without issue. The couch can stay and the cabinets, too. There are three bedrooms, she offers warmly (but one is clearly a storage closet). I imagine it'll be the twins' room—like Kraft Singles, they'll share the same cramped packaging.

My mother says: I think it's perfect.

I ask: Perfect for what?

No one answers me.

The two of them exchange pleasantries and shake hands, strategize about what will stay, what will be taken away, what needs to be signed. I don't understand what their agreement is. I can't figure out what money we're using to buy this new house and why, seeing as we finally have a house and it's not in this remote town where there are no buses and where the churches are as ugly as supermarkets.

I walk into the room that's supposed to be for Mariano and me. I look around and note the shark-gray tiles. They aren't shiny, they don't have patterns, they don't look like parquet, they aren't terracotta. They're just rough—they remind me of reinforced concrete. Covering the walls is a horrible wallpaper with colorful polka dots; it looks like a room for toddlers and swaddled newborns, the restless, annoying ones. You can hear everything through the plaster walls and the room is superhot. The sun beats down on it. It's a greenhouse and I'm a lemon tree.

Knowing I'll be sleeping there with my brother is the only thing that reassures me—to hear him breathing heavily, see him turn off the light, the way he tosses his socks into the laundry basket, how he talks at night while fast asleep, saying: That's enough, horse, moon, farewell, call me, why?

Signora Mirella and my mother hug and my mother says: This house is a lifesaver.

⁓

The first time I see the lake is not the day of the green hat, but the day of the move.

My mother began planning our move well in advance: she wrote lists, found cardboard boxes and tape, and began packing, arranging objects impeccably. I saw her close boxes full of plates and cups as if they were sponges and tissue paper. She carried coatracks and lamps with filial care, and she sweated, cursed, and dragged drying racks, wicker chairs, shelves, all by herself for hours on end.

All I did was what she asked me to do: sort the clothes, put them into piles for each of us, separate the winter things from the summer things and pack, label, and stack the boxes in a corner.

Mariano did nothing to help, in protest of my mother's decision to move, which he found unconstitutional and Nazi-like.

Maicol and Roberto are now five years old, have the same face (only distinguishable by a mole) and with two sets of the same eyes they watch us quarrel, insult one another, and migrate.

When we arrive, the parade of boxes and furniture starts all over again. A friend of my mother's is there to help. His name is Vincenzo and he's known her since they were young. We call him by his name. My father calls him *that guy*.

He has the van, and he also has the strength to lift our meager furnishings and carry them into the new house. He has the skill to get my father up to the correct floor using the elevator, and it's his idea to at least go and see the lake before he takes off again in his empty van.

My mother and I join him. We leave the twins with Mariano, who is wandering around the house like an alien in search of the Milky Way and a stepladder to climb up into his spaceship and disappear.

The Piazza del Molo is full of parked cars. There's an iron railing all along the stretch of asphalt, and I walk onto the pier with Antonia while Vincenzo gets a coffee at the bar.

What's under there? I ask, leaning out toward the wooden pilings and looking at the dark water, which doesn't reveal anything special.

Mud, my mother responds, then adds: Don't look down, look at the view.

I lift my head and she points out the hills and the other towns, the Bracciano castle, the Trevignano waterfront, the woods, Cimini Mountains off in the distance. She says over there is Viterbo, and over there Manziana. She says you can go swimming all along the promenade and all the trees are poplars. She says the water never gets too cold, and I go back to looking down.

But what's under there? I ask again because I saw something sparkle.

Nothing, water, Antonia says and keeps gazing out at the other shores and the other beaches and the other towns. I like the light on the houses here, she adds.

My eyes are fixed to the spot where the phantom gleamed: a shard, a fish, a deflated balloon.

A little blond boy is sitting on the railing with his feet dangling and he points to the same spot, the exact spot I was staring at, and says it's where the sunken nativity scene has always been. There's the Christ child, there's the ox and the donkey. They light them up during the holidays. It's one of our town's traditions.

I lean out and look, then look again, but now I can't see anything. The water is clear and it doesn't reveal the scene I'm searching for.

So I say: I don't believe you.

And he says: Come back and see for yourself at Christmas.

I stare at him defiantly. He's wearing funny little military shorts and looks like he's just walked out of the woods.

My mother pulls me away. She says it's nonsense—a head, an eye, a foot, a robe will never appear in that spot, and I am torn between who to believe: my mother, who sees nothing, or that little boy, who sees everything.

My brother is fifteen when we leave Rome and his nose has grown more and more prominent in adolescence. It's long but has narrow nostrils; its tip points downward, and it has a hump on the bridge. It looks like a steep mountain or the jagged coastline of a northern sea.

His nose is unlike any of ours and it's the only thing his father left him. He doesn't even have his last name or know anything about his biography or occupation. Mariano wouldn't be able to pick him out of a crowd, let alone know how to find him around Christmastime for the customary greetings.

None of us have that nose, which my mother calls distinctive and I call fake (it doesn't look like it belongs on his face but rather like it was left there by accident)—not Antonia, not Roberto, not Maicol, not me, not my father.

Over the years, my father decided that Mariano's nose would be his revenge, a way to make himself unbearable without having to make any big movements. Like a child, he inflicts pain with very little effort.

Every moment is ripe for telling Mariano he has something on his face, something that slices the bread whenever he nods his head yes and clears the table whenever he shakes his head no. The nose comes first and Mariano follows, my father says while smoking on the balcony and ashing into the aloe plant, always seated in the same creaky chair, the shape of his behind well-defined on its stained cushions.

There's an elevator in our new building in Anguillara, and he could take it down and get pushed to the park by my mother or me to sit in the shade, in the sun, to turn sideways, to fall asleep, to be in the world in some way, but he doesn't want to.

His daily route is bed to wheelchair, wheelchair to wheelless chair, wheelless chair to couch, couch to bathtub, bathtub to toilet, toilet to bed, repeat.

Every three days he inflicts the desperate rite of a bath on us and we're forced to help him, lift him in, push him, scrub him, while he curses and cries saying he'll eat us alive. It's always tight for him in the tub, and one time he even cuts his hand by accidentally punching the ceramic soap dish. His blood drips down the side onto the floor; traces of it are still in the tile grout.

He seems to want to make us pay for his survival, as if the fact that he was the one who fell from the scaffolding and didn't die on the spot was damage we caused, our wrongdoing.

Antonia doesn't tolerate my father's jokes, the way he laughs at her son, lifting the corners of his mouth to reveal nicotine- and tartar-darkened teeth.

You don't make me laugh, she always tells him.

Mariano ignores him most of the time, but there are times when he lets fly every possible torment—he insults and hits him, goes up behind his chair and slaps his neck, pulls his hair, and then steps away, yelling: Now stand up and come get me.

My brother isn't very tall, but his body is a ball of nerves. All it takes is a breath of air to get him worked up. He amasses acts of rebellion, from small ones at home to bigger ones at school.

Only fifteen and he's already rotten, my father announces.

Since we left Rome, Mariano has been attending the technical high school for construction management in Bracciano, a town near ours. In the morning, he takes the bus around eight and he's never home before seven. Sometimes his eyes are so red he sees me out of focus, his nose turned into a sharp weapon.

At school, nothing suits him: the teachers' grades are a form of control, the bathrooms are purposefully kept dirty to degrade the students, they force you to play soccer during PE, the history books are full of lies, the computer lab stinks of melted plastic, and the janitors always steal the toilet paper.

Mariano protests each of these injustices.

He speaks in class without raising his hand, interrupts his teachers by discussing books they've never read, conducts sit-ins in front of the principal's office, writes signs he puts up outside of the bathrooms, breaks the vending machines because all the snacks are fancy Ferrero chocolates and they cost too much.

They only feed us things they see on TV, junk from commercials, he claims during dinner, earning himself my mother's tender glances, my silence, and my father's ridicule.

It's your fault he's like this, Massimo tells Antonia. Sooner or later someone's gonna shoot him.

Whose daughter are you?

Antonia's.

Antonia who? Patuzzo's niece?

I don't know who that is.

Then Antonia who? Who are you?

My brother told me lots of things about small towns, like how you have to identify yourself before you can expect any attention, how you only exist once other people have understood who you are, once you've made it clear who your family is, what land is yours—which houses villas apartments—what neighborhood you live in, whether you have a store, if you offer discounts, if you keep your business closed on Thursdays as is customary, whether your brother studies with the son of this or that person, what trade you're in, whether that red Fiat is yours, the one parked right on the sidewalk, or whether you have an automatic gate, if you lower the blinds when a hearse passes.

The people here are obsessed with assigning nicknames; they need to rebaptize you. Everyone who matters is renamed. The name might come from the work you do, the place you live, that story about your grandfather. You could be Fishmonger, Frog, the Train Wreck, and no one will ever let you shed the name the town has given you. It will forever be your tailor-made suit.

In many cases the associations are easy to understand: if you sell bread, you're Flour, if you have a big nose, Schnoz, but for others the logic is not so clear. In fact, nicknames are often inherited from fleeting circumstances, disputes that took place twenty or thirty years earlier and have only survived in the cruelest forms. They're names that leave a metallic taste in your mouth.

They do with you what they do with some places, Mariano says, like Piazza del Lavatoio, where there's no longer a public washhouse; the street behind the Soldati, where there are no soldiers; Via of the Jars; the Cinnamon; Pizzo Bend that juts out into the lake; the Cross.

If you don't know what to call a place, you carry the shame of being a foreigner, nobody's child. They don't know who you'll vote for in the elections, who your family doctor is, what float you'll build for Carnevale, or whether you'll fry lake lattarini at the local fish festival. They don't know how to ask you for favors, so they won't do you any in return. They don't say hello at the post office. They ignore you at the butcher's when you say it's your turn because it's always, no matter what, their turn.

I have to start middle school and my mother tells me that Anguillara is experiencing a boom of relocations from Rome. Houses cost less here, life is calmer, and the train can get you to St. Peter's or Trastevere in an hour. The town is expanding inward and filling up with town houses, paid parking spaces, gas stations, supermarkets, public schools, and gyms. People from Rome are mingling with people who were born here and this mix causes disagreements, uneasiness, anxiety.

They just can't figure out who we are, and the biggest mystery is what led us to their town.

Sometimes we invent believable explanations or outright fantasies—aristocratic aunts, allergies to smog, a love for provincial roads, in Rome you can't even buy fresh tomatoes anymore, we like the smell of cows and ears of corn, we love walking and hiking, one day we'll bike around the perimeter of the lake.

I don't know what really happened between my mother and Signora Mirella. I only know that we have to keep quiet about the details of our childhood. When it comes to our father, we say he's disabled and that's all. When it comes to the house, we say we live there and nothing more. It's not pretending and it's not lying. It's just leaving some things out. My mother teaches us that sharing our family's business, affairs, trivialities around town is much worse than having to face the town naked with our hands tied.

My mother felt we were living like hostages in Rome, and she chose the best solution so that we'd no longer have to deal with certain people, those whose money didn't make them any more transparent to us. The Roman apartment was a pond full of frogs and tadpoles, larvae, earthworms; what we needed was water we could sail upon. That's how she convinced me—with the image of sailboats, of the wind in their sails.

Antonia cleans other people's homes for work, but she knows how to do many other things as well, like how to fix broken furniture, revive slow dishwashers, change light bulbs and bleed radiators, sew simple clothes, patch socks, make budget costumes and disguises, saw wood for shelves and bathroom cabinets. She'll mow the grass when it's long and she has a way with roses. With her enviable green thumb, she maintains flourishing balconies, terraces, and gardens. Before leaving, she always waters the lawn.

Antonia reigns in those houses as she does in ours. She keeps their drawers in order, yells at children, selects detergents, and dictates how to hang out the laundry. She polishes silver with DIY products, comments on slippers left around the house, hates scattered toys, gives every vegetable, cheese, and salami its own container—to which she attaches a label specifying its expiration date. She makes grocery lists that never include processed snacks and Coca-Cola. She combs little girls' hair, giving them braids when they come home from school. No one wants to make her mad.

Other people's houses have multiple floors. Sometimes they have pools, they have garages, they have signs that say BEWARE OF DOG above their doorbells, and long-haired cats on their couches—and their houses are entirely in Antonia's hands.

There is not a single clothespin, cork, washcloth, or remote control that doesn't depend on her, on the nook she chooses for it, on her taste and her tyranny.

The owners place unwavering trust in her: they let her manage their money, they give her the keys of cars that need to go to the mechanic, they pay for her Christmas holidays and August vacations, they give her all the articles of clothing they no longer wear, which she brings home for me and Mariano to try on. She brings them for our father too, who keeps getting shirts that are too large or pants she has to hem for him, even if he only wears them to go, at most, from his bed to the kitchen table.

Over the years, my mother could have stolen jewelry, Capodimonte porcelain statues, silver knives, Swarovski figurines in the shape of little elephants, but she didn't because they aren't hers, and Antonia treats every object that isn't hers with the same amount of reserve and composure as you would treat the dead.

If my father asks her to take something we need, even just as a joke, something trivial like pasta because we've run out, salt because it's all gone, or a roll of toilet paper, she is deeply offended. She coldly declares that she won't be making dinner and, slamming the door behind her, goes out to buy what we need, reminding all of us that what we do and do not have depends solely on her.

It doesn't take long, not long at all, before everyone in town starts calling us the children of Antonia the Redhead.

3

Those Who Have Never
Experienced Pain Are Mean

Growing up is hard work. No one stays a kid for long. You won't be protected, cared for, fed, cleaned, and saved forever. The time will come when it's your turn to take your place in the world—and this is my time.

My mother decides that going to middle school in Anguillara or in Bracciano wouldn't do me any good. Our town is safe, of course, but the schools are better in Rome and no one really has faith in Mariano. The only female child has to know how to study, has to excel, go to university, become a doctor or engineer, go into finance, publish novels, and above all read—compulsively, with no way out.

Many people have spoken highly to my mother about a middle school in La Giustiniana, a busy neighborhood in Roma Nord that's split in two by Via Cassia and has a mix of apartments with concierges and security cameras and prefabricated buildings and Chinese restaurants.

At the school, kids from working-class neighborhoods like Ottavia and Palmarola come together with those from wealthy families who live in apartment complexes with automatic gates and three hundred intercoms to choose from, but it's not where the truly wealthy go. Those families prefer to send their children to private schools.

I don't know if the school ever had a name. I've always referred to it by the name of the neighborhood and of the station where I get off every morning, from the same train that carried me from Rome to Anguillara the very first time. That train has become my means of transit, an escape, a source of frustration—it's always too crowded with commuters, the stations have started falling to pieces, the tickets cost too much, delays force you to sprint so you don't miss first period, and you have to hide from conductors in the bathrooms.

The town is divided into two factions: those who go to school near the lake and those, like me, who take public transportation into Rome. As crazy as it sounds, there are a lot of us. My mother isn't the only one who finds the train convenient and the schools in Rome more suitable.

Every day I get up at seven and wait for the shuttle to the station, which our town finally decided to introduce. At the station I find other backpacks, other noses, other tired eyes like mine heading to school. We mingle with all the high schoolers and middle schoolers, soldiers going from Cesano to Termini, and men with overnight bags who work near St. Peter's. We all get off at different stations.

For the first few weeks I keep quiet, like a larva in its cocoon. In attentive silence, I listen to my faltering thoughts swirl. The train, the windows, and the headrests feel foreign. I'm bothered by the smells of mustiness, early-morning sweat, and nose-tickling deodorants. I sit alone with my backpack on my lap, a backpack that used to be Mariano's and that my mother reinforced with cardboard before giving it to me. After I wrote my name on the pocket and she cursed me; she says Maicol or Roberto will need it next and we can't afford to stain it, draw on it, or turn it into something girly. It was black and it needs to stay that way.

The faces at the station are always the same. Our eyes begin to meet and we even recognize one another at school. Although we're in different classes, we—the kids from Anguillara—are a pack of wolves and lions. We start meeting up during recess, chatting on the train, saying hi in the hallways.

This is how I meet Agata and Carlotta.

Agata is tiny and very blonde. She has a polite smile and light eyelashes. She always complains about not being pretty enough. She's burdened by defects only she can see, yet she attracts all our peers' attention, and not only with her high ponytails and tanned skin (her father has cows, pigs, and pastures, so being in the sun is part of her family duties).

Carlotta's body is ready for womanhood before she is. She already has soft hips, thick thighs, and low-cut shirts. She has a distinct way of laughing—it's almost a whistle—and a tendency to be submissive. Her asymmetrical face doesn't interest the boys, her ears are too big, she has a wide chin and tiny, dark eyes, but she has a self-assuredness that Agata and I—little girls still bothered by our freckles and knock-knees—lack.

I'm not interested in judging whether or not my friends are princesses. We've come together out of necessity. We're three fortified castles—we want an army to defend us, someone to guard the fortress.

We're young enough to not yet be obsessed with our bodies or those of other people, but old enough to sense that the way we look at ourselves and at one another will become a silent war over the years. We'll be on opposing sides, and we'll shoot poisoned arrows at one another's backs.

Is that a new sweatshirt? Carlotta asks.

No, it's my brother's, why? I respond.

It's green like a marker, it makes no sense.

It's what I had at home.

You look like a cartoon character.

Three was never my favorite number. It makes me uncomfortable. I'm used to big numbers, families of at least five, tables where someone is always screaming. I'm well aware that bedrooms are where you go to cry, and I find silence scary.

There's my mother and me, Mariano and me, my father and me. Or rather there is us—the group, the noisy family.

Agata, Carlotta, and I are too few to find solace in one another and too many for me to feel cared for. The three of us came together like some ramshackle thing and it makes me suspicious.

I'm not cut out for friendship anyway. I don't understand the dynamics, the conflicts. I don't know when to respond and when to stay on the sidelines. I can't invite them over to my house, no one can accompany me to theirs. My mother says I'll have to wait until at least next year before I can hang out after school. I'm not exciting. I never have any gossip to share. I don't have toys, I don't have makeup, I don't have clothes to lend. All I have to offer are my brother's sweatshirts, the twins' diapers, my father's wheelchair.

I don't talk about my home life with them. When they complain about the mother who got the wrong gift when she bought a striped T-shirt, or about the bicycle they wanted in pink not purple, I nod. Like a snake that stays belly down in the grass, my latent envy doesn't reveal itself. I cultivate it with care. I keep it at bay at the edge of my gut, feeding it when I'm able, smothering it with the hope that having two friends matters more than being the inferior one in the group.

So I compliment their new tops and necklaces. I get excited when they write affectionate messages for me in my school notebooks. I exchange barrettes and magazines with them (even though I can only buy mine by skipping snack time).

Sometimes imbalances I don't know how to handle are created and destroyed. There are days when they're mad at each other or at me, days when Agata seems to not like me and others when she hugs me tightly, taking my breath away, and invites me to paint her nails on the train; there are days when Carlotta comments on my skirt, saying I look like I walked straight out of a circus tent, and others when she wants to brush my hair and gives me one of her rhinestone headbands as a gift.

Either they have compassion for my shortcomings or they benefit from them because giving to me makes them feel superior. I'm not sure. I think it's a bit of both. I know how to occupy my own space; I learned at home that when you don't spill over into the margins, when you keep to the place you've been assigned—a box, a dresser, under a bed—you won't be a nuisance and you won't stir up dust. Everyone will tolerate you. They won't kick you.

I often apologize to Agata and Carlotta without even knowing why they've lashed out. I prostrate myself before their incomprehensible demands, I follow their unwritten rules, I get behind one of them and then the other. I say *yes* when they insult each other behind their backs; I never side with either of them. I stay neutral during conflicts and wave a white flag when the waters need to be calmed.

I tolerate it because being with them means not being alone at school or in Anguillara. I have our small group on class trips, in the school courtyard, at the train station. We walk into school together and exchange planners to write notes to one another. We talk about the older boys and recount feats and conquests that most often never happened. Together we are witnesses to the tragedy of being small in a giant world.

We're ruthless with one another. We play pranks and steal things that we can't even show off because whoever we stole from would realize. We know we're thieves and enemies but we always come together with the same false smiles on our faces.

We unite when a threat comes from outside our group, we raise our shields, defend ourselves. We lie for one another. We fake illnesses. We go to war against oppressive parents, tyrannical teachers, and gossips.

Our friendship is normal. We laugh, we cry, we take turns winning and losing. Our friendship is stretched like a rubber band, about to snap. It's innocent. It doesn't carry the stench of tragedy on it.

My school has a yellow face with wrinkles and scabs. You have to climb a steep hill to reach it.

There aren't enough classrooms for all the students, so two shipping containers were set up in the courtyard—perfect for the summer mold and winter chill. Each class uses them on rotation, since misfortune should be shared.

There isn't a gym, only a blacktop piazzale, so to have us do physical activity they set aside two hours a week and drew up an agreement with a nearby gym. For half the year, we'll swim in the covered pool. For the other half, tennis in the dome.

We have to pay extra to participate and buy ourselves the necessary accessories: a swim cap, a bathing suit, goggles, a tennis racket.

I spend the first few months of school in a classroom on the third floor. Our program at the gym hasn't started yet, so we play dodgeball on the asphalt for exercise, and to warm up they have us run around in circles.

My friends aren't in my class and I maintain the utmost discretion with the girls who are. I don't confide in them. Some have been held back and are older than me, to them I'm just a childish lump. Others are eager to grow up quickly and do nothing but smoke and sneak into the boys' bathroom. I'm quickly excluded when I say I don't want to join, looked at as if I were a boiled turnip, dinner's tasteless side dish.

I form delicate daily alliances. I don't start conversations. As soon as the bell rings, I dash out the door and look for my friends. I sit with them at what we've decided is our meeting spot, a low wall in the courtyard. My desk, my pencil case, the bathroom where we hold the door for one another, our meeting spot—the things and places we want to mark with our humanity, taking possession of that which is strange or scary.

My friends' conversations are never really that different from my classmates', but I see gulfs and massive waves between them. I swim in my own current.

The boys in my class wear tracksuits and hardly any of them have the polished charm of mature children. They laugh at incoherent, rude jokes, drawing their laughter out. Smiling isn't enough. They spend hours, days, months on the same joke. They're maniacal persecutors. There's one who can wiggle his ears—he's very proud of it—and another so skinny you can see his collarbones through his shirt. One has greasy hair and never takes off his baseball cap. The interesting boys are distant galaxies, always older, in other classes, or in town. Most of them are in town. The people at our school are worthless. You can't classify them and you quickly forget who they are.

My only goal is to not get bad grades, to study on the train, and, after school, show my mother that I do what's right for me. I want to make sure she isn't called in for meetings with my teachers because then she'd have to explain why she's there alone and then she'd have to explain what her job is and then she'd have to explain where we're from and these are all explanations I don't want her to have to give.

The math teacher loves to assign us nicknames, and the one she gave me is pH 4.5 because she says I respond acidly to what she sees as kindness. The English teacher is obsessive and compulsive: If we mess up a verb or a plural, she has us write it one hundred times over in our notebooks. I have pages full of adverbs, pronouns, intransitive verbs. The Italian teacher hates the essays I write. She says I always go on tangents and she loves giving me a D+, a *nearly passing*, with *nearly* underlined in red. Whenever she hears any noise in class she loses her head, closes her grade book, and starts hitting it against the desk, wielding it with both hands. My nemesis is the technical-design teacher because I'm sloppy and never close my circles. I smear all my lines, my straightedge wobbles, and I use Mariano's old art portfolio, which has anarchist *a*'s written or scratched all over it that my mother wasn't able to wash off.

I study like crazy to maintain a passing grade in technical design and do well in my oral exams. I memorize how prefabs and electrical systems, resistant structures and different types of constructions are made. I try to learn everything I can about textiles and ceramics. I show my drawings to my father. He laughs at them and impatiently tries explaining how he thinks they should be done, but neither he nor my mother have done much studying or drawing, writing or interpreting. Or if they have, life has made them forget all of it.

Mariano starts fixing my drawings himself when they're assigned to me as homework. He spends hours turning the compass and using a black ballpoint pen—time that he would certainly rather spend on something else. But we can't fool the teacher. She has me do the same operations again in class and I, as a lefty, smudge all my pages and can't even trace a line that's perpendicular to another.

My struggles in this subject aren't what unleash my fury. In fact, being bad at something protects me. Those who excel at school are the teachers' pets, they're traitors. There's something else about me that everyone is waiting to bite into, like cannibals, and it's my flesh—my flesh that is growing and deforming, stretching, peeling. They search me for the slightest hint of ugliness, any overly tight item of clothing, any blemish on my face.

No one is left unscathed, and no one knows what prompts the cruelty. In my case, all it takes is a bad haircut to trigger guerrilla warfare.

We've never been able to go to the hairdresser. My mother has always cut our hair—the children's and the adults', including her own. The last time she decided I needed a haircut, since my hair had grown too long and was full of split ends, she trimmed it up to my chin, with two much shorter chunks in the front, making my ears stick out. They now look like they're framed by a spongy red bob.

As soon as I set foot in our classroom, my peers notice that something has gone horribly wrong, and they make fun of it. They say I have big ears, that I look like a mushroom, like moss. They call me Little Red Riding Hood and Dumbo. They draw little figures with enormous ears on my desk while I'm at recess and mime airplanes behind my back to make it clear that soon, with those massive ears, I'll take flight.

I examine my ears in the mirror, as I'd done with my mouth as a child, and see that they're the same as always, so I start blaming my mother.

You cut my hair like the boys', I yell at her, coming home from school in tears.

It's not true, she defends herself. Your hair looks very pretty.

I look like a stupid little boy. Now I don't have boobs or hair.

You have both of those things and you're very silly to cry about such nonsense. There's much more in the world besides your hair to despair about.

To you everything else is always worse than what I suffer.

You don't know what it means to suffer, that's the problem, she says. I won't waste my money on a hairdresser we don't need. Use a headband and some bobby pins if you have to and then get back to studying. School isn't about making yourself look good. Antonia ends the discussion and goes straight back to ironing and grumbling. In addition to doing chores in other people's houses, she has to do them in her own.

I run to my room and try to enter, but the door is locked. I knock, then knock again. Mariano is in there with a friend, some girl who says she came over to study.

I think about how much I hate them all and sit on the ground with my back against the door to wait until the friend gets dressed and Mariano decides to let me back in.

My classmates all get bored of me and my ears pretty quickly, except for one.

His name is Alessandro and he's taller than me. He could rest his chin on top of my head if he wanted. He wears glasses with thin frames. He's good at soccer and is always juggling a ball in the courtyard. He has very thick, curly black hair. He changes his gym shoes once a month and his parents own a bakery that makes pastries for the whole neighborhood.

He decides that the teasing hasn't gone on long enough and keeps at it—a lone knight with bronze armor against me, on foot and without a lance.

He calls me Ears. He says it in class, in the hallways, at recess, when school gets out, on the field trip bus. He writes it on my desk and in my notebook. He yells it in front of everyone. He says, Ears come here, Ears do this, Ears go over there.

At first I get mad and complain about it both at home and in class. I try to make sure the teachers are aware, but no one seems to care about my discomfort. They smile at it, shrug their shoulders—it happens to everyone else, so why wouldn't it happen to me.

Then I decide it's best to ignore him. When I hear Ears, I don't turn around. When he walks by, I don't say hi. If I know where he is, I don't go there. If we're called up for oral exams at the same time, I don't help him. I build a wall for protection. I shelter myself, and that's how I trigger him. From laughter comes resentment. From jokes, injury.

One day we're in the courtyard doing our usual warm-up, running in a circle, and he says: Watch out, Ears, or you'll fall.

He trips me and I plummet. I face-plant on the asphalt and hit my chin, which splits open. There's blood on my shirt. Black gravel is stuck in the palms of my hands and my knees are shaking from the surprise attack. I wasn't able to stop it in time.

He looks down at me straight-faced, sees the blood, and has a moment of confusion. He realizes he went too far and extends his hand to help me up. I refuse it and stand up on my own. I head straight to the bathroom to rinse off without saying a word.

Ears, I'm sorry, I didn't mean to, he says from outside the bathroom door. I don't respond.

He tries to save himself by calling me by my real name, but I don't respond to that either. I walk out, and even though my legs hurt, I go back to running in a circle and then I sit in the shade to watch everyone else, including him, play dodgeball.

I see him win and celebrate with his team.

The teacher didn't notice anything, didn't express any sympathy. She teaches PE in tweed skirts and heels. She always has fuchsia-colored nails and wears a beret. She spends more time smoking than running.

That night I tell my mother I tripped over pine tree roots sticking up out of the asphalt.

She replies: I'm going to tell them to cut them.

I say: Please don't.

The episode pacifies Alessandro, but not for long.

Soon he starts up again and even convinces the others to use that name for me, to make the real me disappear forever, creating a new identity: Ears, the thing that's ugly and thin and has no breasts and doesn't know how to kiss and can't draw an isosceles triangle.

He makes sure I'm not invited to any class parties. He gets ahold of my home phone number and calls, says Ears, and hangs up, or he says nothing if he thinks my mother or my brother is on the other end.

He has other people call me, strangers. At night they make our phone ring nonstop, but I don't surrender, I don't tell my mother what's happening, because having her speak up for me would mean admitting defeat.

If I told her or Mariano, they'd intervene and the problem would go away. My mother would start a fight and make a scene and Mariano would come beat Alessandro up outside of school, the kind of thing he used to do. The two of them have the power to make injustices disappear, but this time it's different. I feel more grown-up. I want to learn how to defend myself.

Going to school every day starts to feel like a huge burden. There's no class period without murmurs, without laughter behind my back, without teeth being bared. I feel like a vampire; I have no blood in my veins. I'm always tired and would rather be asleep.

The months at the covered pool begin and make the situation even worse. My mother sews me a swimsuit that's too tight on my butt and that I constantly have to readjust. I have a pink swim cap with rubber flowers on it, like the kind old ladies wear, and my red hair sticks out from under it. My legs are skinny and freckle spotted. I have a chest like a flatfish and unshaven armpit and leg hair. My defeat is clear: this is the end of child me, who neither excelled nor sank.

The reasons to harass me pile up. I bring these things on myself, like my overly large lime-green flip-flops or the fact that I don't know how to swim the butterfly and am always at risk of drowning.

When we return to the classroom, I sit down at my desk like I would at the top of a tower.

All the other girls get their first cell phones for Christmas, they're as big as bananas and gray. They ring one another just to chat. They write ungrammatical texts and call one another BFF.

I'm cut out of this picture, just like with the photo our class took at the Villa Giulia Etruscan Museum on a field trip, where we were bored by the endless crocks and shards and statuettes and display cases. When they give me a copy, printed on glossy, crisp paper, I take a pair of scissors and cut off my head, a little square in the upper-left corner.

Snip, snip and I watch it fall.

The square is what remains. It has Ears' face, not mine. I don't know who she is and I want to forget her as quickly as possible.

I take that face and leave it in my father's ashtray, where I know he puts out his cigarettes without even looking, just as he does this time, after dinner. His ash burns a hole in the photo.

When I see blood staining my thighs, I don't have an angry outburst or any nervous tremors. I go straight to Antonia with my underwear in my hands and my butt bare. I ask her what to do.

She leads me into the bathroom, pulls out her pads, unwraps one, and places it into a pair of clean underwear for me. She opens the wings, makes them stick, and explains that from here on out, for many years, I'll have to perform this ritual.

She shows me where she keeps what are now our pads. They're divided into three groups: the darkest ones for the first days, the violets for when I feel less pain, and the pinks for the end, when it's light.

If there's too much blood, you should tell me; if the blood doesn't come, you should tell me; if you have a bad stomachache at school, you should take a break; if your blood pressure drops or your head spins, you should lie down.

You have to wash yourself, she repeats, even if it makes you squeamish. Take a lot of showers, always use the bidet, wash your underwear and sheets immediately, otherwise the stains will stay.

But the most important thing to know is that this stuff is of your concern alone. It's your responsibility to deal with it. Be careful with boys, even when they tell you to trust them. Even when they seem to understand, they never do. Know that from now on you're able to have children, and not having them is up to you.

Don't end up like me. I had Mariano when I was seventeen with a guy called Tony. He's still serving time in prison for murder.

Does Mariano know that? I ask.

No, and he never needs to. We have enough useless men as it is.

Antonia soaks my dirty underwear in some bleach and I feel a pang in my stomach.

That evening she starts to worry: having me and Mariano sleep in the same room seems clumsy and careless, something to fix.

She arms herself with string and ties it from one side of the room to the other, then sews some sheets together and hangs them up between our beds so I can undress behind them and hang out in my room without being watched.

What is this bullshit? my brother says when he gets home.

Your sister needs privacy, Antonia replies.

A trench is dug between the girl me, who can hear Mariano talking in his sleep, and the woman me, who has to stop doing things like that. Our toys are separated, our clothes are different, posters hang on my side, political flags on his, our beds have mismatched sheets and pillowcases. We're shadow puppets. I see him appear and disappear behind the fabric, like a marionette.

My body really does change, and everyone is concerned about it except for me. My father starts showing unfamiliar jealousies and anxious impulses: who's talking to me, who's calling me, who are my friends and my enemies.

He's made a habit of paging through my notebooks and diaries whenever he's able to get his hands on them and he worries that I'm unfledged in the world, without a father protecting me.

It never struck me as something he'd be afraid of, but ever since I began shedding my skin like a snake, he's started asking Mariano to keep an eye on me. He tells him: Watch your sister, see what your sister is doing, where your sister is going.

Mariano says he's not my babysitter and they start yelling.

Everyone fights and hurls insults at one another over meals, but the worst fight of all is the one about the tennis racket.

The pool months at school are over and we're about to start tennis lessons, but I still don't have a racket because we haven't found a used one and they're too expensive to buy new.

My mother, who has sensed my darkening mood, insists that we buy a racket, so she reallocates the money used for things such as my father's and brother's cigarettes, electricity and telephone bills, cleaning products, and her hair dye.

What will she do with tennis lessons, huh? My father gets worked up at dinner, across from the boiled carrots and stracchino cheese. It's wasted money, straight down the drain.

Massimo, the lessons aren't the point, my mother responds, slamming her water glass on the table, making it spill. All the kids at school are doing it. She needs a racket and she needs it now.

He's right, what is this shit? my brother chimes in, strangely on Massimo's side. She's not even thirteen. She might play tennis twice in her life.

Now that I'm a woman, they've remembered that they're men and have formed a new, unexpected axis alliance.

Maybe I haven't made it clear that I'm not asking for your permission, my mother looks at Mariano sharply. I'm just informing you that I'm putting money aside for the racket and each of us will be making sacrifices to buy it.

Are you gonna do that for each of us? Will we all have our own rackets? I want one too. Mariano gets heated with a piece of bread in his mouth.

Don't even try with me, you're not getting anything. Your sister is going through a tough time. I know this, as her mother, and you, as her brother, should understand. Instead you're always out bumming around and doing your own thing, meeting people, making your rounds. You think we haven't noticed, that we haven't figured it out by now?

Tough how? Because she has zits and no ass? You think that's tough? You're such a hypocrite.

I'm the one helping you all get by, you're nothing without me. My mother stands up, throws her plate on the table, and it breaks. The carrots splatter, the checkered tablecloth gets dirty, the twins cry.

I am the candle and the wax. I remain extinguished, balancing in the candelabra.

But within a week I have my tennis racket and they've stopped talking to each other, as usual. Antonia took something crucial away from Mariano: her words and attention.

Tennis lessons begin and I feel like I have to follow along very carefully. I'm always sure to put my racket back in its case. It's one of the first things I've owned that's new and all mine. I feel responsible for it.

After every lesson, I go home and tell Antonia what I learned: how to serve and stay light on your feet, the balls I hit, the laps I ran on the red clay.

I don't like tennis, but I revere my racket. I gaze at it tenderly. I paid the high price of having to sit and listen to Mariano being unfair and my mother condemning him for it. Of course I have to take care of it.

Being in the dome and playing tennis is certainly easier for me than swimming in the pool. My tracksuit isn't pretty, it's neutral. It isn't noticeably weird. It doesn't have patches or flowers on it, and my racket is the cheapest of them all, but it's shiny and clean. I carry the case over my shoulder proudly and flaunt it at the train station. I show it to my friends. It's new, I say, brand-new.

They have cell phones and pierced ears with pearl earrings, but I have my racket and I don't care.

Until the day it's broken.

My indifference toward Alessandro has grown in step with his cowardice. His face turns red with rage whenever I don't look his way. He feels ineffective, like someone degreasing an already-clean surface.

He gets crafty and, like a mosquito, bites where he knows there's skin. He brings a pair of shears from home, sticks them in his backpack and, while I'm splashing my face during a quick break, cuts the strings of my racket, severing them as though they were veins.

There's a hole right in the center, making it useless. He hides the shears, puts my racket back down on the bench where I'd left it, and goes back out on the courts, overlooked by distracted teachers and complicit classmates.

I find it mutilated next to the bag where I keep my clean shirt and change of underwear. Its snapped strings have taken away its power. It's flaccid, ruined, defenseless—an oval object with a pointless handle.

Alessandro flashes a headstrong, gleaming smile at me and I know he did it.

The matches and training sessions resume but I can't play anymore. I sit on the bench. I feel zapped, drained; my thoughts are racing about the money it'll take to repair the racket, the time it'll take me to tell my mother about it, and how I'll be seen as a fool because I didn't protect it.

I stand up at the end of the two hours and approach Alessandro.

Can we talk? I say.

About what, Ears?

About the racket.

No.

Did you do it? I show it to him—broken, punctured, destroyed—and he shrugs.

In the meantime, all the others have left the dome, and our teacher asks us to gather up the cones and yellow balls since we're the last ones there.

Did you do it? I repeat, ignoring her.

Now we're alone.

Maybe, he grins.

To him it was only a bit of mischief, a harmless game, a pinch in the belly, a push on the swing, a pull of the hair.

I think about him and the watch around his wrist worth three of my rackets, his gel-filled curls, and the moped he's been promised for his fourteenth birthday. I think about his name-brand T-shirts and designer glasses, about how delicious the zabaione-filled pastries his mother makes are, about the candy-pink frosting. And then I think about the checkered tablecloth at my house, the broken plate, the carrots, the discount detergents, Mariano—who now hates me and only sees me from behind a curtain—the German lady who wouldn't let me play with the fish, the gates the Fascists stole, Antonia making the gesture of sticking a syringe in her arm, the cardboard box where the twins had to sleep, my father in intensive care without the use of his legs—and I start to strike.

I raise my racket up high by its handle, I grasp it with both hands, and I give it to him on his knee, one time, two times, three times, five times. At the seventh, he falls to the ground and screams.

Blood gushes from his wound. It ends up on the brick-colored earth. He tries to stand and can't. I throw out my bloodied racket even though I know that if I'd just told the teacher, she would have gotten it fixed and called his parents in for a meeting and they would have apologized, but it's too late for that now.

I leave him there with his broken knee and walk over to his bag, unzip it, pull out his racket, and slip it into my case. I don't tell him that this is a fair trade. I don't demand an apology or his atonement.

He curses and screams and gasps and I exit the dome. I walk briskly down the gym's steps to the street, the gas station, the train-station piazzale. I sit on a bench with the racket over my shoulder and wait for the train, the 1:23 toward Viterbo Porta Romana. I spot Carlotta and she asks me how it's going.

I say: The train will be five minutes late.

Maybe it's not the roses you snatch from public gardens that turn you into a bad woman, it's not the library books you don't return on time, it's not all the moments you eat with your mouth open, it's not the emergency lanes you use to pass, it's not the fights with children over fruit gummies. It's not the lies or the bad intentions that turn you into a bad woman, it's doing violent things like this.

4

The World Is
a Cold Swimming Pool

When I was a girl, the square of concrete that my mother had made safe for Mariano and me was the only place we could play. Our elementary school had no yards or soccer fields. We had recess in the hallways because a pine tree had fallen in the courtyard, getting in the way. They'd roped off the area with red-and-white tape to show that it was off-limits for the children, and no one ever removed it. Whenever the tape broke, someone would just tie it back together. For five years, from my classroom window, I saw the trunk of that tree weighed down with needles and pine cones, its roots rotten because of the concrete. It lay lifeless across the courtyard, as though telling us its death was a sign of our mistakes.

The parks near our first house were full of syringes, and even during the day, women and men would sit on the benches with their arms outstretched and needles still stuck in their veins. They'd forgotten to remove them, and no one bothered to do it for them.

Whenever Antonia saw this, she'd approach, saying: Somebody get that thing out of his arm, somebody, please, and I'd feel like crying out with anger. Those people could've attacked her, mutilated her, forced her to carry their burdens. I was afraid of them and felt no compassion.

My mother made a rule that we could only play at home—just me and Mariano and no one else. There were no swings or slides, no open spaces where we could ride bikes and bump into other kids.

Antonia was afraid that by going out into the world we would come across the same kinds of games she had played when she was young, in deteriorated places that weren't meant for children.

One time she told me about the neighborhood she lived in when she was a girl, about the day posters were put up saying construction had begun on a public pool where there would be swim classes for neighborhood residents and affordable prices for the elderly and for children. The city government promised new facilities and bus lines, emptied trash bins, and a decrease in drug dealing.

Work began on the pool. They dug it out, bulldozers and cement came, then engineers and safety-and-compliance plans, then the mayor and the assessor—everyone came to see something no one would ever finish.

The pool was built, but it was never opened. The concrete was poured, the pool was insulated with resin, the diving boards were installed. There was never any water.

With time, the public pool became a specter of itself, a farce and a mockery. It was supposed to be the neighborhood's rebirth but instead became its surrender. People began filling it with trash and furniture they no longer used: mattresses, broken armchairs, cracked bathroom tiles, exhaust pipes. Instead of chlorine, people poured in insecticide. Instead of life jackets, there were mice and cockroaches.

And yet in that expanse of stuff no one wanted anymore, in that stench of neglect and carelessness, the kids went to play just the same. They had nowhere else to go. There were no parks or piazzas, and they made sure not to go to church. My mother and her friends used it as their meeting spot. They'd say to one another: See you at the pool.

The pool contained the sewage of broken promises. Kids would sit on the diving board with their feet dangling over the disease-ridden heaps. They played hide-and-seek among the skeletons of what would have been the locker rooms. They smoked behind the large tarp banner where it still said: NOW OPEN—PUBLIC POOL.

The tarp showed the time and place—it had everything on there—but the pool had never opened. The paint was peeling from the rain and the tiles had fallen off. The contracting company had declared bankruptcy; it was under investigation for various offenses, but then the investigations stopped. Procedural documents were stacked on top of other procedural documents. It was a pile of inefficiencies, of dead things.

My mother told me that was when she stopped believing, when they said that they'd clean up the neighborhood, they'd help those who had been thrown out on the streets, they'd give houses to families without work, they'd build a new playground, a new tram line, a new local health department. She had mocked them.

Antonia stopped waiting for things to get done; she started doing them herself. Her children wouldn't be playing in the puddles of that lost mirage. If there was something that needed to be cleaned, she would clean it. If there was something that needed to be prohibited, she'd prohibit it. If there were boundaries that needed clarifying, she'd clarify them.

When my mother sees that they're setting up carnival rides in the piazzale right across from our house in Anguillara, she interprets it as a sign of all the sound choices she's made. Maybe she's forgotten how forbidding children's games can be, that at fairs and carnivals, in order to win a goldfish or a stuffed elephant—the most coveted prizes—you have to take aim and shoot.

The carnival comes to town once a year, during the Easter holiday, and it stays for a couple of weeks. On one end of the piazzale, they set up several strange silver spaceships that move up and down. They have red snouts and look like rockets. Mainly little kids ride them, dragging their parents over and pointing their fingers in the air, imagining the ride's mechanical, repetitive movements as an experience of flight and the unknown.

Then there's always the swing ride: chairs suspended with chains from a rotating top that, once set in motion, start spinning faster and faster, higher and higher. The way to win the game is by pushing the swing in front of yours hard enough to help whoever is in it reach up and grab a prize that's usually hanging from a pole. It can be a simple game for kids if the ride is spinning slowly or a devilish competition if spirited teenagers are playing, like us, or at least like we want to be. We're still twelve, neither fish nor fowl. We think the spaceships suck, but we don't have mopeds or money for cigarettes.

There are three attractions we like best.

The first is the boxer, a machine with an oval punching bag hanging from it. The stronger your punch, the more points you get. The boys can spend hours, entire days competing for who gets more points. Some have a running start, others hold their elbows up high and furrow their brows. If you don't move the bag by at least a centimeter, you're a loser who'll be put to shame by everyone else. We girls stand around in a circle and watch them win or lose; we cheer or we laugh. We sneer at their beardless, sexless virility and encourage them to man up. Whoever punches the hardest is treated with respect. It's like he's the mayor, walking with his chest pushed out. The girls aren't allowed to try, but we wouldn't want to even if we were. A woman who fights and injures falls from grace. She's not desirable. If one of us approaches the boxer, we do so as a joke. We give it a soft tap, which doesn't even earn us half a point. Our punches are worth the same as an infant's.

The second attraction is Carlotta's favorite: the bumper cars. In the middle of the piazzale, right below the balcony of my house, a black covered track is set up. Inside, cars with two seats and worn leather steering wheels zoom around in circles. They each have a number painted on the side, and the only fun thing about it is making the cars crash because they have thick rubber bumpers on all sides that soften the impact. But bumping into one another is not enough. In fact, we target one another. The boys survey the situation from afar and take wide laps. They spitefully seek out cars to crash into. Every collision makes a *crack* sound, and when their cars touch they trade insults. But this isn't why Carlotta likes the bumper cars, a family-friendly ride that we've colonized, making it unfit for the little ones. She likes them because the ride operator came up with a new variation: the kissing game.

At some point while you're driving on the track, the operator sounds a siren and all the cars stop; then a number is called and the person in that car has to stand up and go kiss whoever they want. The person who receives the kiss wins a token they can use to go again the next round for free. The fact that you can win with kisses thrills Carlotta, who always chooses Agata to be her carmate since she gets more kisses than I do. I remain a ghost. The mere possibility that my number could be called stresses me out and makes my fingers sweat. I wouldn't know who to go to or what to do. It goes without saying that among the boys there are certain faces I like more than others. There are people who I'd want to choose me in front of the other girls, one boy especially. His name is Andrea. He's tall and his hair is cut evenly across his forehead. He speaks without much of a dialect compared to the others, often wears colorful T-shirts, has round eyes. A lot of us like him. He knows how to carry himself. He responds when he's insulted, he doesn't hold back when he's called upon, but he's not aggressive. He's never the one to start an argument.

Simply imagining him climbing out of his car and walking toward me when his number is called makes me tremble, but he never does it. Whenever his is called, he has his friend stand up while he stays seated. I can never tell where he's looking, if he's looking at me, if he's looking nowhere at all, if he's thinking about something else, who he's thinking about, what he's laughing about when he's whispering with his friend.

Carlotta loves to stand up and choose who to kiss. She does it with a sense of ease that I hate. The angst of expectation never gets the better of her. She's always ready for any challenge, any opportunity for growth, though the boys don't appear particularly happy when she chooses them. There's something in her, maybe in her face, in her unkempt eyebrows, or in her widening hips that they don't like.

I'm embarrassed by how eagerly she offers love no one wants. I turn away when she's the one standing up, and the only way I know how to protect myself from all the kisses ungiven and unreceived is to keep driving my car around in circles and selecting who to take it out on—speeding up and crashing into someone, harder and harder, hard enough to propel their bodies forward, twist their necks, contort their backs. I get more satisfaction seeing the lost look in the boys' eyes when a girl slams into them than the look of flattery on their faces when a girl gets up to kiss one of them. I'm wearing my baggy sweatshirt and have the hood pulled up, covering my hair, ears, and half my forehead. Sitting there, I'm just like them.

Why are you so angry? Agata asks me when the round is over. She's won four tokens. She could spend the rest of the night there, whereas I've already used up the money Mariano gave me that morning. I have nothing left, so from now on I'll just be watching from the sidelines with all the other unlucky kids.

I'm not angry, I say. That's how the game works. It's called bumper cars, not kissing cars.

I use a tense, shrill tone of voice that I barely recognize, but that I feel has become part of me, seeped into my bloodstream, ever since I won the racket war with Alessandro.

Since that day, Alessandro no longer speaks to me and he never had the courage to tell anyone that it was a girl who beat him up. Our teachers investigated. His parents were outraged. They sought damages, said they'd press charges against the school. Their son had to go to the emergency room. He'd no longer be able to play soccer.

Want to shoot? Andrea says, and I look around to see who he's talking to. I don't respond.

Want to shoot? he asks again and pulls some money out of his jeans pocket. He's talking to me.

The third attraction that fascinates us is the shooting gallery: empty Coca-Cola, Sprite, and Fanta cans are lined up along a wall, already dented. You're given a BB gun or rifle. The more you knock down, the more you win. Three cans gets you nothing. Ten gets you a toy frog, mouse, or giraffe. Thirty earns you a fake spumante bottle full of chocolate candies, and if you knock them all down, they give you an enormous stuffed animal: a pink bear, two meters tall, with a red bow around its neck and black eyes like a jellyfish.

I've never played. I think it's silly, a money grab. I'm sure most of the cans are glued to the wooden supports. So yes, you can knock down up to thirty, but no more. I've seen people try, and no one has gotten more than the number necessary for a handful of chocolates, which they then went off to eat, sitting on the wall, before returning with their jeans covered in chocolate and tobacco.

I gawk at Andrea and say: Okay, let's try it.

He pays for the first round and starts shooting. He has a crooked grip on the gun. He takes aim too hastily. You can tell he doesn't know a thing about weapons, that at most he sits on his living room rug and invites his friends over to get killed in video games. I don't think real guns should be held as if they were carrots, broccoli, eggplants— as if they were inert—but instead with an awareness of what you want to shoot.

I watch him hit a few cans. Some he only grazes, others don't even budge—almost all of them stay standing. His friends come watch. Even Carlotta and Agata cheer for him. Although we've never been introduced, we all already know one another. In our town, if you've ever spoken to someone, if all you've done is approach them, that's reason enough to band together.

Andrea says it's my turn. He puts more money on the counter and I see a flicker of challenge in his eyes. I guess what had previously seemed like an act of kindness is meant as a practical joke. Seeing as I'd crashed into him in the bumper cars like someone with unrequited love, with a hunger to be understood and accepted, now I have to suffer.

I pick up the gun and the woman at the shooting gallery stall tells me how many shots I have. If I want more, I have to pay more and would also have to start over. One round, one prize.

I accept. The people who'd been watching have all walked away. No one cares to see the little girl with the hair badly cut by her mother, wearing her anarchist brother's clothing, shoot and miss. Maybe I could make them laugh, but even laughter isn't worth much if I'm the one who's causing it.

When our Italian teacher saw Alessandro return to school on crutches, her eyes filled with tears. She murmured with a hand over her mouth: Things like this shouldn't happen.

I take the fake gun, raise it slowly and, when I close one eye and aim, I have neither the shivers nor a racing heart. I feel like shouting: Look at me, now I can play, too.

I start shooting and the cans start falling. You can hear the clinking of the tin and the blanks—five in a row fall and I stop. I rest my hand. I don't know how I did it. I felt my stiff arm, my finger pulling the trigger, my eyes focusing on the target. It was as though I had sung out loud for the very first time and discovered I had the voice of a nightingale.

Andrea is on edge. He tries making a joke about luck, about how he thinks there's wind. He laughs.

I raise the gun again, aim at the sixth can, and shoot. I knock down five more and reload. The shooting-range woman, with her greasy hair and low-cut, gardenia-pink dress, smiles tightly and says something in a dialect that isn't ours and that I don't try to understand.

There are people who can balance on one foot like flamingos, people who have rhythm when dancing and can feel the beat of the drums, people who don't need paper or a calculator to add or subtract. And then there's me, a girl who knows how to shoot and has rough legs and a big sweatshirt and no thoughts about her unknown future.

The mere fact that there's something I could win makes all the difference to me. It might not mean much to the others, but for someone like me—who wants to accumulate things, who wants piles of shoes and lipsticks and hair ties—that enormous pink animal with its ears and round nose represents accomplishment and reward.

I raise the gun. I see the cans clearly—one, two, three. I keep shooting. As a kid, I never got to go on a carousel and I would've liked to dress like a princess, put a crown on my head, hold a scepter in my hand. But rides cost money, crowns cost money, glass slippers cost money.

Only one shot left. It feels like a lot of people are standing behind me now. I've attracted an undeserved and unhealthy amount of attention. They're saying: She's just a girl, she doesn't even have arm muscles, she doesn't even have the money to buy new underwear.

I'm going to be like one of those people who gets close to the finish line and then trips. I'll be the loser in the photo finish, the horse that gets injured in the final curve, the bucked-off jockey, the soccer player who screws up the penalty kick, the fourth-place medal. When you lose narrowly, you lose because your emotions take over, you get distracted, your own human nature gets in the way.

I shoot the last shot, the Coca-Cola can wobbles, and I realize there was no scam: they've all fallen. I set the gun back on the counter.

My friends scream. They can finally say they're friends with a hero instead of that homely girl who should be left on her own at the bumper cars, the girl they call Ears at school, who wears T-shirts the color of highlighters.

But I don't feel any happiness. There's a part of me that's still locked in, frozen, shooting.

I look up at the can lady, who's staring at me.

I want the prize, I tell her, and stretch out my arms. I'm ready to embrace the world, the entire universe.

She turns around and struggles to get the two-meter-tall bear out of her stall. She disappears behind it. She doesn't know how to give it to me and I don't know how to receive it. It's almost twice my size. It's a person, a giant. She puts it down on the ground in front of me and says: Congratulations.

She says it joylessly. She's confused by what she's just witnessed, she wonders whether I cheated and how, who actually shot the gun. I'm unsure myself. I debate whether or not to turn around and check if anyone's there.

But in the end I look up at the mass of fur in front of me. Maybe I should hug him or give him a name. Maybe I should leave him there, say I don't care about him.

Thanks for the money, I say to Andrea, who doesn't know if he should be surprised or dismayed.

It's called beginner's luck, he tries to say and stares up at the bear. He feels like it could fall over on him. He wants to laugh because I won an absurd prize that he doesn't want, but for some reason no one laughs.

I don't know what else to say, and I see Mariano walking into the piazzale to look for me. It's already nine o'clock, time for children to go to bed.

What is that? my brother asks.

A bear, I say. Help me carry it home.

Mariano looks at all the kids nearby as if they were plants or rocks, and without saying another word he takes it by the head, I take it by the feet, and that's how we get it up to the apartment, where we push it through the door and drag it into our room where it'll be impossible to hide.

My mother has the radio on. She's listening to music, singing Patty Pravo to my father while he smokes near the balcony. Neither of them knows there's a pink bear in the next room.

But the following day my mother sees it there by the curtain separating my half of the room from Mariano's. She stands and stares at it, asks where it came from.

I won it, I explain.

And how did you win it?

At the carnival. It was the prize for winning a game.

What game has something like this as its prize?

The one where you shoot.

She's silent and then catches fire. Her jaw clenches. Her eyes button up.

You must take it back right now.

No, I won it.

I don't believe you and you don't need it.

Everybody needs it.

No, no one needs it, it's a pink bear. What a perverse, cursed world where they let children shoot guns in order to take a stuffed animal home.

I yell that she can't take it away from me and I slam the door in her face. I want the whole house to shake. She keeps yelling that shooting shouldn't be done as a joke and it shouldn't even be done for real. I don't listen to her. I look at my prize. It's big and expressionless, like a sphinx.

It's the summer of 2001. I've finished middle school and left behind the math teacher who loves to assign mean nicknames. I've forgotten the tennis courts and the too-tight swimsuits in the pool. I keep the racket hidden in my closet. I didn't make amends for my mistakes. I still don't know how to draw straight lines or circles with a compass. I have no clue about what's happening in the world. I live in limbo between my downfalls and my unpredictable triumphs.

My childhood is now only a memory of heroines in skirts, dancing puppets, snack commercials, and MTV music videos whose existence I discovered on other people's screens. I saw these images by accident or when, finally set free by my mother, I was allowed to go over to my friends' houses and spend hours engrossed by all that was forbidden to me while they chatted without paying it any mind. They were used to the constant rotation of tops, exposed midriffs, and pop-star microphones.

The truth is that I'm thirteen years old and still haven't had my first kiss and it's July. The end of the month is almost here and another battle is being fought in our house: my mother has pulled out her shield, Mariano his sharp sword. They're in the middle of the living room, about to challenge each other to a duel.

My classmates are taking a train, my brother explains.

You aren't going anywhere, you're only seventeen, my mother says. The twins are sitting on the floor, competing to see who can collect more dust.

I am going, actually. People are coming from all around the world to protest. The train is leaving from Termini early in the morning . . .

You aren't taking any train, and this is the last time I'm saying it.

You don't care about what's happening? They're financing fake wars, all they think about is money and their investments. You don't give a shit about the banks, about the money we owe them? You of all people, who don't even have a house of your own . . .

You're saying a bunch of things you don't even understand. What do you know about wars? What do you know about banks or owning a home? All you should be worrying about is studying, working, and not getting yourself arrested.

You don't understand.

No, you're the one who doesn't understand. You're seventeen and you aren't going to Genoa. You're staying right here where I can see and hear you, where I've decided you'll stay.

Aren't you the one who always wants to save everyone and go on strike? I thought you were against any and all subjugation.

I'm the one who is older than you and who has seen much more. I know what I'm doing, you don't. You're a child.

I'm still going. You can't keep me here.

My father tries to get a word in: Antonia, we've protested, too. We've spent time out on the streets. The kids need to see what's happening, they need to be on the front lines.

Oh yeah, they need to? Look at us: you without your legs and me mopping other people's floors and wiping their asses. The kids need to study, that's it. Times have changed, those political days are over.

They're over for you, Mariano presses.

I have the same look on my face that I do whenever life passes me by like a freight train. I have no idea what they're arguing about. My instinct is to plug my ears and scream. I hate this family, its defects, its torments.

Mariano tells my mother she's a loser. He spells out L-O-S-E-R so she understands.

A few days later he gets up in the morning and pretends to go to a friend's house but instead takes the regional train and then the metro, then he gets to Termini and boards the train to Genoa.

We don't have cell phones, we don't have a television, we don't have a computer. We have little means to communicate with. We're locked in the past of a world that's galloping forward. It overtakes us, crushing us beneath its hard hooves.

My mother uses our home phone to call Mariano's friends. She calls their mothers, their fathers, and their teachers on vacation, asking everyone: Who gave him the money for the train? Who told him which platform to go to? Who is he traveling with? Where will he sleep?

Antonia turns on the radio and listens to the news at the kitchen table. She has the machine glued to her cheek, as if she doesn't want to part with it. She's like the shadow of a child locked in the cellar of a bombarded building.

He'll be home tomorrow, Antonia, you'll see, says my father the grouch, the detached, the nihilist.

Shut up! she screams back. Her voice is shrill, it passes through the walls. You're the one who's been going on about the piazzas and the protests. You told him to go. It's your fault.

Their yells overlap. A voice in the background crackles out from the radio saying the situation has changed, the demonstration has taken a turn and now chaos reigns, now people are afraid. The police have started to intervene. The voice reports who has fallen to the ground, who is escaping. The voice says *black bloc, families, squats*. It offers confusing details and eventually says that a boy has died, then repeats *black bloc* many times over, then *fire extinguisher*. My parents shout over each other that this time it's really over, they're breaking up, they'll separate their lives forever—you here, me there, you need treatment, it's about time you get on antidepressants, you're a poor cripple, you're completely out of your mind.

Fear washes over me. This only happens to me within these walls. This is where I cultivate all my neuroses. We have no news of Mariano and it feels like he's already gone, swallowed up by the cosmic churn.

My mother stuffs some things in a backpack and yells that she's going to get her son back, wherever he may be. There's no policeman, no gathering of powerful people, no army that can keep her from getting him back.

We're pathetic, she screams at my father and hurls a half-empty glass of wine at him.

It hits the elbow he'd used to cover his face. By now she's all impulse and destruction and she shows no signs of stopping. She is blind to the twins' wide eyes and indifferent to the fact that I'm watching all of this unfold, standing motionless next to the cold radiator. It's as if I'm seeing her through a bubble of clear water. She appears to me refracted, altered.

Antonia really does go to Genoa, she really does retrieve her son, she really does bring him back home. It takes some time, tires her out. She travels through places I've never heard of. She speaks to people I've never met. She doesn't tell us how she did it. She never talks about it.

The house awaiting her is now a fault line, an open wound, a burst abscess, a scalpel that has cleaved flaps of skin.

I tended to my father's arm while he stared silently at the tiles behind the sink. I made meatballs and dressed the salad, put the twins to bed, waited for the night to pass while sitting on the toilet (when I'm nervous I have to pee constantly), and slept hugging the sink for two hours. Then the next day I started all over again, and the day after that, too. I'm good at shooting and cracking kneecaps with rackets, but my family is my weakness. I can't fight against them.

Mariano comes back looking like he's been in the trenches. My mother asks him to gather his things, and to be quick about it. She says: I will never go through another scare like that. You don't deserve to be my son. You don't deserve anything.

My father and I don't understand what's happening. We thought the whirlwind of events was over. We thought the sutures were set.

Take your things and go to your grandma's in Ostia. I'm done dealing with you. My mother chases Mariano with her voice and pulls his shirts, socks, wool hats, and cigarette filters out of the drawers, all under the dead gaze of my enormous, pink stuffed animal. The bear is enjoying the debacle and seems to smile at it, like he already knows what will become of us.

If you're such an adult, if you're so good, then actually grow up.

I know Mariano wants to throw himself at her feet, apologize, and beg for forgiveness. I know because I see how his eyes are darting, fiery with anguish. We're nothing without her. Who knows where we'd be if it weren't for her. But he doesn't do it, he doesn't put his hands together and beg, he doesn't tell her she's right or that it's true: Genoa was too much for him.

My father shifts around in his chair, his elbow bandaged, his face covered in sweat. The heat of late July is making him melt, and he keeps saying: Antonia, this is bullshit.

But Antonia doesn't listen to him. She makes clear that this isn't a two-chamber parliament. There's no balance of powers. This is her domain.

Massimo watches Mariano pick up the bags Antonia packed him. He carries his future under his arms. After years of bitterness, side-long glances, violent words, years of *this boy is just like you* and *this annoying kid* and *this little brat*, Massimo appears to be suffering as Mariano exits the scene.

Maria', please don't go, Massimo calls out with the confused, dense air of a foggy morning.

Antonia ignores him and accompanies my brother to the door.

My brother looks back at us for a moment: me, my father, the twins.

My father's frustration is evident in the way he grips the wheels of his chair, well aware that he can't stand up and do something. Powerless, he watches my mother make her decision.

The door clicks shut, my brother leaves, the curtain of revenge and alienation falls on us.

A few days later, I ask my friends if they saw anything about Genoa on TV and they say no. The *Dawson's Creek* reruns were on. Joey likes Pacey more than it had seemed.

I smile and say, Of course, as if I were some sort of trout, a whitefish.

July is ending. I'm hurtling into August on a bicycle seat while someone else pedals.

Only a privileged few have mopeds. We ride around on bicycles that people were given as birthday gifts. I don't know how to ride a bike, I've never owned one. So I found a boy who does. His name is Federico. He's shorter than me and has a symmetrical face. He chivalrously comes to my house every afternoon, loads me onto his seat, then pedals standing up to the spot we chose for our summer vacation, with all the others, the nontravelers, the exiles from schools in Rome and nearby towns.

We call the place where we meet the piazzetta, but really it's just an intersection of a few streets in the Residenza Claudia neighborhood, the part of the residential area within Anguillara that stretches from the train station to the road that leads to Lake Martignano.

The piazzetta has no special appeal. There's just a lamppost to sit around and avenues for doing wheelies on. There's no bar or newsstand, no pool hall. Our meeting place isn't near the lake. It belongs to the new part of town.

There are few points of interest around there: a hotel pool that charges an entrance fee and where they have swim and water polo classes in the winter; private farmland full of hay; and an abandoned house that's been vacant for years.

Agata and Carlotta claim that Federico loves me with the kind of passion you'd struggle uphill for, and that he'd sacrifice friendships and stability for me. But I don't feel anything for him besides gratitude, so I keep him at a distance. I place my hands on his hips only lightly, and once we reach the piazzetta, I speak to him sparingly, with little enthusiasm.

Federico is Andrea's friend. He and a few others chose the piazzetta as our stronghold and gathering place. They bring stuff to smoke and spend hours talking about the soccer-championship finals. If someone has a ball, they kick it around a bit, but their favorite thing to do is to go to the abandoned house.

I still don't have any awareness of my sexuality. I've rubbed against my pillow in bed for reasons I don't understand: constellations of images from Mariano's magazines, conversations heard on the street, advertisements. I have a weak imagination and my experience boils down to having seen my brothers naked, with total indifference and no sense of its import. My parents haven't had sex in years and none of us care to investigate this lack. Today they're less close than ever before, but they still support each other through their shared yet opposite pain.

The only person with clear thoughts in this respect is Carlotta, who tells Agata and me about the inquiries and proposals she's received from the local boys. Her eyes widen with a nauseating sense of triumph.

Agata and I know that our ignorance is embarrassing. We distance ourselves from what is unfolding all around us. We don't have the vocabulary, we don't understand how it works, we float along at the end of childhood with our flat bodies, without breasts and without butts. We're basically mannequins.

Agata is more interested in Carlotta's stories than I am, stories about Francesco, about Vincenzo, about Lorenzo. Every day she adds another name to her collection of been there, done that.

The most I can bring myself to confess is my interest in Andrea. He's still the only boy who gives me goose bumps and makes my heart beat fast. Several months have gone by since the day at the carnival. I haven't told him or my friends anything about Mariano being thrown out. I haven't mentioned the cold war being waged within the walls of my home. Andrea seems to have a kind of respect for me that often keeps me at a distance. I'm not who he turns to for cigarettes or money to borrow. I'm not who he rides around on his bike. I'm not who goes with him into the fields to crush pine nuts with rocks as if they were maggots.

Rumors, accusations, lies, whispers start circulating about Carlotta. The names of the boys she's shared her body with keep growing: the just-touching boys, the hands-between-the-legs boys, the unzipped-jeans boys, the get-on-your-knees boys. Where once there were two, now there are twenty, thirty. It seems like all the boys in town have seen her naked. She's pleasured every one of them. She's satisfied them all.

On one of the many nights when Agata and I sleep over at Carlotta's house—all three of us crammed into a full-size bed—we listen to her detailed stories of intimate things we know nothing about.

When we ask how it's done, she says: It's easy. You sit behind him and reach your hand around and touch.

Then I open my eyes to the ceiling and see the posters on the walls—the pop singers, the actors, the sunken *Titanic* and Jack who wasn't able to save himself—and I think about how we won't be able to save ourselves either.

Carlotta insists that I should offer myself to Andrea: They never say no if you ask to touch them. I tell her that I can't. The truth is that I don't want to, but I don't know how to explain myself.

But if you sit behind them, that means they never look you in the face, I say, and my comment lingers in the air.

One afternoon soon after, Agata and I sit under the lamppost in the piazzetta for hours, waiting for Carlotta. She was supposed to be there at four, but now it's six o'clock and she's nowhere to be found. Federico warns us that she went to the abandoned house with five boys. Who knows when they'll be back.

Agata says: Shut up.

I'm not ready to face such judgment or put in any effort. We should be getting up and joining her in that house to touch, lick, indulge along with her, but we don't make the slightest movement in that direction. I feel like concrete. All I want is solitude, my repressed desires.

When Carlotta comes back from the house and one by one those five boys also emerge—some we know, others we don't—she has a satisfied yet twisted smile on her face. It's the same way a comedian might look at the end of a show, ready to go cry backstage because the audience didn't clap enough. Her initial feeling of success, which had made her feel appreciated and respected, is starting to dim. It's tinged with new colors.

I stand up and set off down the road toward the abandoned house, where I've never been before. I want to see what's inside, what revelations about our growth, what rites of passage, what oracles.

I find myself inside a simple two-story house with broken plumbing fixtures, used condoms on the ground, empty beer bottles, empty cigarette packs, cigarette butts, cans of paint. It smells like a sewer. Some people drew on the wall, wrote their names. I find Carlotta's. She put a small red heart next to it.

The walls of the house reverberate with misunderstandings and trapped bodies, with unmet expectations, with undeveloped breasts and cellulite in thighs, with low-rise shorts that look awful on that saggy belly. You're thirteen already: go on a diet, cut out gelato and candy, eat as little as possible, until you vanish.

August will be over next week and we're saddened by the realization that this summer can never be repeated.

High school, classes, classmates, decisions await us.

We all decide to go to the hotel pool to celebrate our final days together and spend the day jumping in off the diving boards, bothering the patrons with young children, and licking Magnum ice cream bars while sitting in the sun with our legs crossed. Federico sees me rummaging through my empty change purse and generously pays my entrance fee. I mumble a thank-you. I wish someone else had come forward, one of my friends.

I'm wearing a two-piece swimsuit Agata lent me and it feels scandalous. I walk around with a towel around my chest and only sit in the shade. I quickly turn watermelon colored anyway. I see Andrea calling me over. He wants to throw me into the pool, but I shake my head.

I've been sleeping horribly the past several nights, contorted, with my knees bent, my neck stuffed into my shoulders, my jaw tight. Even though the sheets dividing our room are still hanging, my brother is no longer there on the other side. When I called him from the phone booth he told me: It's so hot in Ostia.

Our bodies are cold in the house, moving stiffly from one room to the next like snowmen. I don't want to get caught up in the numbness. I keep that feeling securely locked in the confined space of my family memories.

I'm lost in my thoughts and find myself sitting in the sun. The shade has moved elsewhere. The others are splashing in the water, running along the edge of the pool, diving in. I submerge myself, too, because it's so muggy, but I get back out right away. The chlorine reminds me of middle school and I don't want to think about all of that. I quickly recover my towel.

I look around. I can't find Carlotta, so I ask Agata where she went. She tells me she's showering and that she wanted to go home. I ask Federico if he's ready to leave, too, because I feel worn out, drained by the heat and my helplessness. He says sure and that he'll wait for me outside.

I gather my things, including the eucalyptus shampoo I stole from my father. I hold the little bottle in my left hand and my brush in the right, dripping while I walk, leaving a trail. In the locker room I call out: Carlotta?

I hear a shower running.

I brought you some shampoo, I say.

Then it gets quiet. The shower stops. Two people are whispering, and I'm reminded of all the things I still don't know how to do— how to offer myself, how to touch, how to find pleasure.

The shower door opens and Andrea exits first. He slips out without looking at me, adjusts his bathing suit and grabs his towel, tying it around his waist. We're in the girls' locker room and I still have my brush in one hand, the strong-smelling eucalyptus shampoo in the other.

Carlotta walks out of the same shower. She holds up the top part of her swimsuit with one hand and says: Here I am.

I'm standing still in the same spot, and so is Andrea. We form an uneasy triangle. I wish I hadn't followed my instinct to come look for her. It's like when I know my father has gotten his wheelchair stuck under the table, or one of the twins has wet himself. I have a sixth sense for when things are off.

I don't respond to her *Here I am*. Instead, I turn around and walk straight out of the locker room and away from the pool just as I am—with my wet red hair, blue flip-flops, and my feet awkwardly sticking out. I'm still holding the shampoo and brush. I start heading home. Federico sees me and asks what happened. He's ready to leave. I don't respond.

I've suffered an affront and deep within me am trying to figure out the best way to react, how to aim the gun at the target. She knew I loved him. She knew about my inabilities, the silences, the misunderstandings. She'd heard me declare feelings that were, in my eyes, definitive. If I hadn't gotten up, if I hadn't gone to the showers, she never would've told me. She was committing a crime behind my back.

This first betrayal feels like an assault, and I suppress my feelings, trapping them between my eyelashes. I don't let them turn into tears. I compress them, as if I had an industrial press or a pair of pincers. The heat of my disgust flattens the betrayal. I walk quickly toward home, still wet, still holding the brush, still the smell of eucalyptus, and still the *flip-flop* sound of my sandals.

My parents are at opposite ends of the table, staring each other down, casting jinxes and spells with the power of their thoughts. I'm still sopping wet and off-balance. The sun went straight to my head, and now everything's spinning. I take two steps and slip. I crash to the floor.

Just a few days later, in New York, the Twin Towers fall too.

5

Melologue

Summer ends and my mother discovers the four books I checked out from the library—two are in the bathroom and the other two I keep on the bedside table in my room.

She's leaning against the washing machine, leafing through one of them, turning the pages with distaste, flipping back and forth. The cover is bright pink with a green embossed title: *This House Is a Disaster.*

Who is Linda Romsey? she asks, mispronouncing the name. She repeats it three times and keeps getting it wrong. Her back is still turned to me. I'm barefoot in my pajamas, standing outside the bathroom door.

I don't know, the woman who wrote the book, I say. I feel my stomach grumble.

And who's ever heard of her? What does she write? My mother waves the book around, holding it by the spine. She shakes it, as if trying to make some hidden secret fall out—something that might reveal who I really am or what my purpose in this world is.

My friends are reading it too . . .

What are you doing with a book like this? She raises her voice and turns around. You've spent the entire summer wasting time, that's what you've done. You really want to go to a classical high school? Do you have any idea what liceo classico would've meant to me? I couldn't even dream of going to high school. I only made it through middle school. I taught myself everything. I'd see girls my age still wearing backpacks when I was already working at an old woman's house, washing her stairs, and after a few years, I got pregnant, had an abortion, got pregnant again, then Mariano was born. This house is a disaster? I had you get a library card so you'd read the kinds of things you should be reading. Instead, you'll go to your high school and tell them about Linda whatever, some unknown writer, and these brightly colored books. What are you, eight? Did you even ask the librarian for recommendations like I told you to?

Yes, but she gave me really hard books . . .

Ah, so that's how you are. When things get hard, you abandon them. You spend your time doing things that are pointless, just like everybody else.

Mamma, it's just a book for passing time, I say, pointing at the one she's still holding.

Books should not be kept in the bathroom; they aren't hair salon magazines. Time is already slipping away, my dear. The summer is over and you haven't read a thing. You want to study Latin, you want to study Greek? This house is a disaster?

My mother slams the book down on the washing machine, only because it's the library's and not ours. Otherwise, I know she would've cut it to pieces, would've swallowed the pages, would've used it to wipe up the sauce that had spilled on the floor. She turns toward me, with the look of someone who does not let things go.

From now on you need to show me every book you check out from the library. You really want to go to the liceo classico with your friends? Then start studying. School is a privilege; you won't be able to keep lying around belly up. Either you study or you're a nobody. Understood? Do you want to be a nobody?

I stay quiet, thinking about the librarian's round face, her uneven, shiny bangs that she doesn't wash enough, her fingers with bitten nails, the colorful rings she wears, that blue one on her thumb. I think about the books she hauls up from the basement, up and down, up and down, and the list she handed me when I asked for her advice— because my mother wanted me to read serious books, real books, the kind that give you chills, make you cry.

I saw one around the house a while ago . . . by an English author, what was her name? my mother keeps going, undeterred.

Jane Austen, I say, feeling my feet burn as I stand in a scalding puddle, soaking in the soup of our words.

How hard can it be? They even made a movie out of it! she shouts, and my book looks like a corpse in her hand, something dead and monstrous. She presses her fingers into the cover, tracing its errors.

You never read it, I try to defend myself.

It doesn't matter if I did or not. I'm always working—do you know what it means to work? I doubt it. All you do is complain, that's what you do. You're a thorn in my foot.

I go back to being passive and mute, and in the silence I hear the low hum of all the books I might never read. I wonder why she persists, what she wants for me, what she's planning. I wonder if it has anything to do with my brother's absence, whether my insignificance has become obvious, if she's trying to fill me up at any cost, like stuffing a bra, a quail, or an overcoat.

Are you even listening to me?

Yes, I'm listening to you.

You look like a dead fish. She stares at me, straight through me, piercing me from my stomach to my kidneys.

If you don't get at least a B+ average at this high school, you won't be leaving the house anymore; I'll lock you inside. Your father and I are about to spend a lot of money on schoolbooks. You'll have to pay me back.

Yes.

We'll read together if you don't understand. I'll study with you. We can do it; we have to. Her voice quivers while she opens the washing machine, grabs the wet clothes, and pulls them out. She's still working to pay the machine off. My mother hates mixing darks and colors, but she also hates wasting water. She turns off the faucet while I'm brushing my teeth and gets irritated if I'm in the shower for more than ten minutes.

Her *we* feels like a prison, it's a *we* I was never even asked to join.

I chose a rich-kid high school. It was an act of self-punishment, like a deep cut or suffocation. I picked a challenging school where they teach dead languages no one speaks, and I tell myself I did it for my friends. They're going there and so am I. But the truth is that I carry something so very small inside me, the size of an acorn or a bug, that guides me—it's the voice of my mother, to whom I always have to prove my worth.

Her invisible *we* reigns over me, creating castles in the sky and swamps on Earth.

On the first day of high school, I learn that walls crumble even in the places where the rich go to school. The courtyards have roots that tear up the asphalt, and the gyms stink of ancient sweat.

The building has three floors. It's a brick red rectangular prism surrounded by stiff and sparse pine trees, parking stripes, and a soccer field. The basement houses the volleyball court, the wall bars for climbing, a worn pommel horse, and rings that hang from the ceiling like salami and prosciutto. The lucky classes are on the top floor, where they can watch the boys playing soccer from their windows; the unlucky ones are down in the basement, next to the auditorium, where it's colder and the walls are made of plaster (they fall apart when you punch them). Everything smells like mildew and moss down there. Sunlight filters in, distractedly and at an angle.

That's where I start my first year: in the cellar, like a rodent or a roach.

At this school, like the last, I quickly discover new shortcomings: I stand out for my shortness of breath and my aversion to volleyball sets and spikes. I wear terry socks that are too big at the toes and tracksuits misshapen at the knees. I'm always cold, tired, and hungry for approval. I have a desperate need for no one to forget about me, a desire to introduce myself and say over and over: Here I am, here I am, here I am.

The walls, inside and out, are covered with graffiti: insults about the most feared teachers, crossed-out declarations of love, stolen phone numbers. Cracked shells and stains can still be seen on the school's facade from the eggs people threw at the end of the previous year.

This school is also on Via Cassia, but it's farther away, so in order to get there I have to take a bus—the 201—in addition to the train. The last stop is at the south entrance to a residential area called Olgiata, where there are tennis courts, golf clubs, villas worthy of the Imperial Fora, maids and gardeners, guards at every gate: the very rich outskirts.

I have to get up at 6:00 in the morning to be in class by 8:20. I barely eat breakfast. I gulp down milk and a couple of cookies— my stomach is tight. The trains are worse than ever, like cattle cars, with people breathing on the automatic doors and shouting insults at every jolt. There's not even room to sneeze. Once I get off, I often have to run, my bag bouncing on my back, because I see the 201 arriving on the other side of the parking lot.

The bus has few seats. It passes slowly by my middle school, which now looks tiny, withered, and limp, like a plant at the end of winter. Because of all the stoplights, there are some stretches where it's impossible to imagine going faster than thirty kilometers per hour and others where suddenly the road clears and the traffic seems to flow like blood in clean arteries.

But sometimes that's not enough. Some days we're stalled and are forced to get off in front of the detour to the Grande Raccordo Anulare highway and have to walk the rest of the way to school. On this route, I weave in and out of exhaust fumes from the backed-up cars and notice an altar—Agata points it out to me. It's enclosed by a fence, with a bouquet of fake flowers at the center and two photographs framed in rusty metal. Someone tells us that's where two girls died years ago when they were riding a moped and crashed into the lamppost. It feels like an omen of some future regret, having to pass by this spot for the next five years of my life without ever knowing them, and imagining myself there too, in a photo on the side of the road, as the river of indifference and the rush to get somewhere flows by.

Agata and I are in the same class, but Carlotta changed her mind in the end. She preferred a local high school over the one in Rome, so she's going to the liceo classico in Bracciano, near where Mariano used to go to school.

Ever since the incident at the pool, I've offered her no explanation— only coldness and silence exist between us. Whenever someone mentions her, I blurt out mean things and spit on her name as if it were a spider or ant, a bug I could drown. I know full well that every word of my contempt will reach her, so I weigh them down with sharp-edged rocks. I'm not above insulting her or ensuring her destruction.

When she says hi, I look the other way. When she walks past, I bounce on my toes like a boxer, ready to throw a punch. Carlotta keeps trying to get closer to me, to slip through the cracks of the wall I've built, but I brush her off, like she's flaking plaster. I reject her, vomit her out.

I don't ask her who she's spending time with, who she's dating, how it's going at her new school. I ignore her stories and get irritated when she complains. I rejoice when she's struggling. Every word that comes out of her mouth is a lie, a clumsy attempt to get noticed and find a way back into my life. I try to shove her back into the hole of her shame. I keep replaying the image of her stepping out of that shower, holding her towel. I can still smell the eucalyptus and feel the bristles of my brush digging into my palm.

Being in class with Agata makes it easier to leave Carlotta out. She'll never be able to join our conversations about the new world that now belongs to us. On the rare occasions when the three of us are together, she'll linger on the outskirts of our gossip and stories, and I'll pretend she's a ghost. I'll emphasize things that don't concern her. I'll bring up specific anecdotes from school, with ample details. I'll act like I'm only talking to Agata, but I'll use a lively tone, a voice that doesn't sound like mine—making things up, boasting about other people's wealth, stressing how close we are to it. It's something Carlotta will never have, but we will, because when you're within reach of money, you inhale its scent. Luxury is contagious, I say to myself and to her, without looking her way.

The truth is, as soon as I step on the bus, I can feel the tension in the air. The girls wear strong perfumes, like they're adult women going to work in some office, and in the winter, the boys wear coats stuffed with goose feathers and wool hats with the brand names showing—they all look so alike you can barely tell them apart. Among them, the kids from Olgiata and Le Rughe—both areas in Roma Nord with three-story villas, front and backyards, pools with diving boards, Persian rugs, and closets the size of entire rooms— recognize one another at first glance. They know they won't be taking the bus with us for long, just until they're old enough for mopeds, and then minicars (those tiny cars that sound like tractors but can be driven before you're eighteen). Me without a bicycle, them already behind the wheel. Soon we'll be looking at one another from our parallel universes, the Milky Way between us.

Even Agata, who has never lacked a thing and has always been able to afford luxuries that are out of reach for me, limps along behind that endless parade of disposable fashion.

For us, even imagining new Nike or Adidas shoes is difficult, and while they come to school wearing Prada shoes and carrying Gucci bags, crammed with notebooks and pens after shopping sprees on Via Condotti for their birthdays—we continue to use the same backpacks we had in middle school.

When my mother and I went to the stationery store to buy school supplies, I pointed out a black Smemoranda planner. She glanced at the price then told me we'd be making my planner ourselves, with two small notebooks, just like we do every year. All we had to do was divide each page in half, write the date and day of the week, and leave space for assignments.

Standing frozen in the greeting card aisle, surrounded by rhinestones and pictures of puppies with wet noses, I almost screamed at her that I wanted a real planner, not a notebook with the days written in it, not a calendar, not another rip-off. In response, she tripped me, her knee behind mine. Then, ignoring my outburst, she went ahead and bought the notebooks she wanted, the pens she wanted, the pencil case she wanted—pale pink and too long.

My new school rejects me immediately, like I'm some expired condiment, like thawed and refrozen food. In response I dig in and anchor myself with my worn-out backpack and a notebook in place of a real planner. I build a barricade and prepare to fight—when I see battlefields, I begin to march.

My red hair has grown back, long and symmetrical, making my face look thinner. I always keep my ears well hidden now, shielded. I don't dare put my hair up in high ponytails or buns. I don't have breasts, I don't have a butt, but I'm thin, and I start wearing the few fitted clothes I own, showing off my ribs and skinny wrists. I covertly apply mascara on the train, and when I look at myself in the mirror, I feel like I'm coming out of my shell—I have to be ready to become my best self, to leave behind the low opinion others have had of me.

There's only one thing that can save you if you don't have money, and that's beauty, I tell myself, brushing my hair more often, pulling down my cheek to draw eyeliner on my lower lid to darken and enhance it, make my eyes an object of interest. I only have a few things, but they won't make me look like my mother—the disheveled one, the laborer, the dishwasher, the woman with the linen suit from the street market that she wears to pretend she's someone she's not. I have to stop being a flawed little girl as soon as possible and transform myself into a woman to love. I'm itching to change. I plunge headfirst into the fierce contest of bodies and gazes.

A week after school starts, I tell Federico that we should kiss—I need this baptism. There will be no do-overs and no applause. We won't go to the abandoned house, and we'll never meet on his bicycle again. To me, he's like a cod fillet, the kind you keep in the freezer for emergencies, for when there's nothing else to cook for dinner.

The kiss goes badly. It's more like chewing and munching than a sign of affection. Drool pools at the corners of his mouth and he's shorter than me, his hair reeks of gel, and his kindness is a nuisance.

It happens behind a wall in the piazzetta, neither hidden nor in plain sight, under the pine trees that drop caterpillars all over the ground.

Federico asks to see me again and I wipe my mouth with the back of my hand. I don't want any trace of my unspoken plea for help.

I say: No, I'll be busy, and turn my back on him.

Our subterranean classroom makes all of us students feel like nocturnal creatures. To stay awake, we flutter our eyelids like moths.

Agata and I sit together at a middle-row desk. In front of us are the overly studious kids; behind us are those who want nothing to do with books. None of them, I'm sure, feel the same pressure that hangs over me: the need to keep my grades above a certain average, so as not to rouse the three-tailed dragon dwelling in my mother's chest.

There aren't that many boys, and almost all of them are ugly. I keep telling Agata that in every other class there's at least one decent-looking guy, but not in ours. One blushes whenever he speaks and his hair is fine and sparse. Another is short and stocky with a face that's too big. One has oily hair and mole-covered skin, and another is known for his overlapping front teeth and misshapen nose. I'm repulsed by all of them. I want to bury them underground, or scatter them to the wind.

Only one redeems himself, but he's out of the question for other reasons. His name is Samuele, and he's already flunked twice; he's the only student in our class who's repeating the year. He's not yet old enough to leave school, so he keeps failing with willful neglect. He has the face of a child: puffy lips, eyes that are both sweet and sinister. He often wears tracksuits and tattered shoes, but certain details reveal him as the son of affluent parents—his watches, bracelets, and gold chains.

His shoes are worn, yes, but he gets a new pair each week, destroying them while playing soccer in the afternoons. He doesn't bring a backpack to school, always shows up late, sits in the front, and either sleeps or reads the newspaper or books of his own choosing, none of which are part of the curriculum. He instills fear and awe in us clumsy and awkward first-years. In class, he often rolls cigarettes or softens hashish to smoke a joint during break, and the rest of the time he ignores us as if we were all frogs and he the prince. At the sound of every bell, he escapes to meet up with his ex-classmates or upperclassmen, who act as school representatives and will soon be heading off to university.

He scares me, Agata says to me one day.

After all, Samuele had arrived an hour late, stinking of alcohol because he'd drunk two beers first thing in the morning. He's wearing a yellow sweatshirt, his eyes are swollen, and he slurs when the English teacher tries asking him about the homework, saying: The moon fell last night, the world's about to end.

The rest of us stay quiet; a charged, reverent silence fills the room.

Our Latin and Greek lessons are torturous. The teacher is strict and exerts a powerful authority over us—she doesn't even need to raise her voice. Her disapproving looks descend on us like the night; she could make us disappear simply by uttering our last names. Even Samuele respects her—during her class, he always dozes off without causing any disturbance. She doesn't even acknowledge him, she treats him no differently than the fern in the corner.

For the first few months, we're all bewildered by these languages we don't understand and don't want to understand. We repeat declensions and verbs like robots and dolls—at home, on the train, in the kitchen, before, after, and during lessons. We drag ourselves around with dictionaries under our arms, each one weighing as much as a bag of flour or a bottle of olive oil.

My Greek and Latin dictionaries are old and filthy. We bought them used, from a friend of my mother's. The pages are yellowed and the margins are filled with other students' incomprehensible notes, leaving no space for me to pencil in conjugations for written tests, for whenever those dreaded Greek translation exercises show up on our desks.

I find myself asking, What am I doing here? while leafing back and forth through my dictionary. I remind myself nobody speaks this ancient language anymore, not even in Greece.

My first grades are barely passing, assignments marked in red pen that I don't dare show my mother. I hide them and forge her signatures in my planner—while for the others a C is reason to celebrate, for me it's a disaster.

Now that Mariano's in Ostia, Antonia focuses all her attention on me, assigning me all the chores and responsibilities I used to share with my brother: from washing dishes to cooking, from ironing clothes to making the twins' beds. I'm constantly helping her with this and with that.

Finish your chores and then go study is her daily refrain.

There's no more going out, and the opportunities to see my friends are rare. I've already forgotten how Federico tastes, and Andrea is a taboo subject, the curtain has closed on him.

My mother hunts me—I'm the fox, she's the rifle. But then, one day when I come home from school, she, smiling, surprises me with a brand-new Italian-language dictionary on the kitchen table.

She says she asked Signora Festa, whose house she cleans, what would be a good gift for a girl who loves to read. And with exacting cruelty, Signora Festa had replied: A dictionary.

This way you can compare words with Latin and Greek. I really wish I'd studied languages. Isn't this great? All the words, all in the same place . . .

Antonia opens the dictionary at random and points to a page. She sets her glasses on the tip of her nose, and says: *Melologue*, which comes from *melos* and *logos*, you get it? The things you're studying. A text accompanied by music—read this for me.

She tosses the dictionary into my arms, still smiling, her eyes shining with a dream. So I look where she'd pointed her finger and repeat: *melologue*, and then I read the entire definition out loud.

My mother's joy clings to me. After so many months of her dark moods and curt words, I can't bear to make her sad, so I flip through the dictionary and pick another word. And in this way, we remain suspended in the moment, absorbed in what we're learning. With every term I pronounce aloud, she comes alive and repeats it, trying to make it hers, with the accent she will never shed. There's a dynamic force driving me to chase her satisfaction, pushing my own aside.

Since she gave me the dictionary, my days have become full, my studying compulsive and destructive. I never stop. I don't think I'm any smarter than the others—I just apply myself. I eagerly pursue grades: from a C to a C+, from a C+ to a B, from a B to a B+. When the Greek teacher hands me back an assignment with an A written on it, I jump to my feet.

The others stare at me, speechless, and then they snicker, but I don't care. I've seen them playing with their cell phones under their desks, passing notes during lessons and tests, and peeking at other students' papers, all while Antonia's words rattle around in my head: So that's how you are—when things get hard, you abandon them.

I don't even tell my mother about the A because a single grade is like knocking down one can on the first try—I have to keep shooting until there are no cans left standing. I want to go home and show her that I don't just bring back useless prizes—gigantic pink bears, gummies, chocolates. I'm a source of pride. I don't give up.

By the time I do well on a third assignment, in different subjects, even in math, my classmates start to notice my skills and they don't know how to react. I'm not repulsive enough to be seen as a smartass, but I'm also not rich and apathetic enough to be challenged or confronted.

They begin asking for my help before oral exams, requesting summaries and advice. During written tests, they stretch their hands out toward my paper and peek. I try to help Agata, who I know is falling behind, despite being studious—I think she has learning difficulties but she doesn't ask for extra help. But when Samuele strides over to my desk as soon as the Italian teacher leaves the room and violently snatches the paper from my hands to see my answers, I don't sit back and let it happen. In a flash, I'm on my feet, snatching it away: Go back to your seat, I tell him, my eyes steady, my voice firm.

He looks down at me, his wiry figure towering, his eyes narrowed into slits. He's not used to having people tell him no.

You're just a poor bastard, a nerd covered in patches, he sneers in dialect, putting my misery on display, accusing me of it, making it clear to everyone that I'm the only kid from a poor family in our class. He underscores that I'm a guest, an intruder, someone who somehow got incredibly lucky.

I don't respond because the teacher walks back in. Agata touches my arm as though to comfort me. She's expecting tears and a lack of composure, but I brush her hand away and focus on smoothing out my crumpled-up test. I rub it up, down, and sideways, while glaring at Samuele's back.

My mother has a basket full of patches—scraps of fabric she sews onto our clothes to reinforce pants, mend pockets with holes, repair frayed seams, and cover burns or stubborn stains on shirts.

At break, he's the first to leave the classroom, and I follow him. He's taking the stairs, and I take them too, going up two floors behind him, then all the way to the top. I see him disappear onto the terraced roof where access is prohibited.

I step out onto the roof as well, the cold, clear Roman sun hitting my face. There are other boys out there with him, all older than me.

Only then does he notice me and my red hair.

What do you want? He turns toward me with an unlit cigarette in his mouth, nervousness and derision in his eyes.

And as has happened to me before, images start flashing across my mind—my struggles and conflicts, my despairs and ambitions, all the things about me that have never been respected or understood: the library and my mother's threats; pages upon pages of pages by pages; her smiles when she repeats *melologue*, *melos* and *logos*, music and words; Tiziana the librarian's bangs; the list of books without which you're nobody; everything I was forced to read while everyone else was reading books to pass the time, for leisure, for fun; the hours of studying while my parents shouted and fought; the books open across my knees on the train and in the bathroom; the sunsets I miss because I'm stuck inside; the grades that rise, that fall, that judge me. These thoughts fuel my desire for war and for revenge. The time of being defenseless is over. I've learned a few things by now: I know how to shoot, I know how to fight, I know how to punish, and I know how to kiss.

I close my hand into a fist, and with the frantic force of my fragile body—with my protruding hip bones and the audacity of someone who has always had to struggle for everything, I punch him square in the face, hitting him in his right eye. Samuele staggers backward, bringing his fingers up to his injured eye, and with the other he looks at me, mystified. Despite his half blindness, he tries to see if there's someone else behind me—but no, there isn't.

You're the poor bastard, you understand? You're the poor bastard—you can't even write in Italian. You don't scare anyone. Daddy's boy, I scream and spit and my saliva gets on his shoes.

I don't know if my intensity was enough to hurt him. My knuckles are aching, burning, my tendons and muscles are quivering, and my eyelashes are wet from the fury, from the rage that rose up inside me. I had to let it out, and now it's back in the world.

My rage is stretched out on the roof, sunbathing and making faces. She slinks among the shadows and looks over the shoulders of whoever is near. My fury is vicious and alive—she has a face, hair, and hands. She wears ripped jeans and carries a leather bag over her shoulder. Her absurdity and mismatched clothes make her stand out. My anger is excessive; she has long legs, small ears, hairy feet.

When she's around, I usually go home—not to the one in town, but to my true home—the one Mariano and I drew on the concrete when we were kids, our H-O-M-E. I sit inside it, within the lines we traced.

I'm sitting on the tuff-and-concrete wall next to the soccer field. The PE teacher told me I'm lopsided and that I have the stamina of a mollusk, the strength of a shrimp. He made me run around the school three times and all I got out of it was the feeling of going in circles without ever reaching a destination, a safe haven.

The kids in the other class are playing soccer. Some brought their cleats from home, others are wearing jeans and sweaters. They're having fun kicking the ball high above the field so the light makes it dazzle and impossible to dodge—it's a boulder falling from the sky.

Are you crazy or what? Samuele sits down next to me with his hands in his pockets and I don't respond.

Not everyone is like me. Sooner or later, you're going to get yourself in trouble. His slightly red eye doesn't seem to have suffered much from my aggression. I hate that I didn't leave a scratch.

You don't even know what trouble is, I say, after thinking about it for a few minutes.

He looks at me, and there's no anger or accusation in his expression—instead he has the face of someone who's been caught in a lie. A boy who brings books from home and reads during class can't be an imbecile or indifferent—he never needed my answers in Italian class. It was just his way of attracting attention.

What's that guy's name? I ask, pointing at a boy on the field with longish hair that flips at the ends, since Samuele isn't saying anything else.

I don't know, he responds and pulls out a cigarette, pinching it between his index finger and thumb as if trying to crush it.

Yes, you do. I've seen you talking to him.

What, now you're spying on me?

No, I'm spying on him.

Samuele stands up and clenches the cigarette in his fist: Then go ask him yourself.

When he walks away, I don't follow him, I don't apologize. I refuse to back down from my own overblown behavior.

The boy's name is Luciano—I've already asked around about him. I know where he lives, and I know his moped's license plate number. I found out he has a huge house with three floors and two yards, his mother wears Louis Vuitton, and his father drives a wide-hipped Mercedes. I know he's going to grow up to be a real estate developer like his dad, and he'll receive jewelry on his birthdays. I know everyone at school likes him, even the older girls—they write him notes and slip them into his backpack, scrawl his name with hearts and arrows on the whiteboard during break, and bombard him with their phone numbers and pleas for attention. I stand up from the wall and walk toward the fence around the field, watching how he laughs and how he walks. I think to myself: Rich people walk like bards and knights, like soldiers.

A few days later, during break, I tell Agata: Wait for me by the coffee vending machines, I have to take care of something, and I disappear among the students crowding the atrium. I go out into the yard and spot Luciano sitting on the wall. He's not smoking; he's downing an apricot juice. I approach him in front of his friends, say ciao, and introduce myself like we're at some conference or a masked ball—I try to keep my cool. No giggles, no innuendos.

Luciano's holding his juice in one hand, the box green with two illustrated apricots intertwined and a no-added-sugar notice on it. He looks at me with the sly eyes of a hunter. He squeezes my fingers with the other—his grip is generous but not friendly.

We exchange only a few words. I'm wearing a black skirt that used to be my mother's, held up with a hidden rubber band because it's too big on me, a pair of dark tights rolled down at the waist, gym shoes I bought at the flea market last Monday, and a large gray sweater. My translucent face shines, my freckles are like stains, and my hair looks unnatural.

So I'll see you at the movies, I say, not as a question but as if confirming something that's already happening. He says okay and asks if I have a phone number. I tell him no, no cell phone—just a house phone. A wave of shame washes over me, breaking around my stomach and rising to my throat, but I hold my breath and swallow the humiliation down like asbestos dust.

Luciano stifles a smile but still puts my home number in his cell phone. He has me repeat my name because he's already forgotten it. I think about the photo finish race I'll have to win, scrambling to answer every call before my mother does and asks me who is this and where does he live and what does he do and what's his family like— as if our family was the gold standard.

I say goodbye and not much more. I don't know what excuses I'll come up with to go to the movies, how I'll even get there, or how I'll pay for it. I don't know who I can tell that I've never been to the movies, except for that free showing of *Mamma Roma* in the piazza one summer. It's Antonia's favorite movie, but it only made me anxious; I fell asleep halfway through just from the stress of watching it. I don't know who I can tell that we don't have a television, that we live off radio dramas, serialized novels in magazines, and books—all things that are singing their swan songs and dying off.

As I head back inside, I hear my name being called from above. I look up and see Samuele peering over the roof as if he were going to jump. I ask him what's up, but he doesn't reply, he just retreats behind the parapet and disappears, his shadow no longer looming over me.

That afternoon, I tell Agata that I'm in love—but it's a lie. It's nice to lie about love; claiming I know something about it validates me, makes me feel like part of an orderly cosmos. I tell her not to mention it to Carlotta, saying: She knows nothing about love.

We aren't very close to our other classmates—we only talk to a couple of them. They live in Cesano and travel with us on the train, sharing space and time. We're slowly starting to see them as potential confidants. One is named Marta, and she gets exceptional grades with disarming ease, which makes me bitter and upset. She doesn't seem to have to work as hard as I do for recognition. The other is Ramona, she's the daughter of a military man. She has Neapolitan roots. At school, they often tease her about how she pronounces her *e*'s, but she has a special talent: she can laugh about almost anything, except for blood. One time in class, when she cut her finger on a piece of notebook paper, she took one look at her hand and fainted.

I tell them too, about this first feeling of mine, already analyzed to death, studied like a specimen under a microscope, and completely artificial, like a prosthetic replacing a limb lost to a grenade.

From that day on, I keep them updated on Luciano. They think it's unlikely he'll reach out, but I wait, making no new moves. Then one afternoon while I'm studying geography, our home phone rings and I leap to answer it, anticipating his voice. Luciano tells me there's a cop movie playing on Saturday that he'd like to see (he doesn't seem too concerned with what I want).

I say that I was interested in seeing it, too (even though I've never heard of it before), and we set a date at Ciak cinema on Via Cassia—a place I can only reach with two buses and a train—but he doesn't need to know that. I don't think getting to know each other will be part of our date; I'll have to put on an act whenever I'm around him.

Smile and nod like a little girl. I like your house, I like your mother, I like your car, I like the way you kiss, I like you naked, I like this movie—it's exactly the one I wanted to see, how'd you know?

With Marta's help, I tell my mother I'm going to study at her house in Cesano, and I take the train right after lunch. I'd asked my father for some money and disclosed the movie plan to him, playing the trust card to make him feel involved in my life. But I left out the part about a boy, because whenever he hears talk of men—now that he can't rely on my brother's strict supervision anymore—he gets anxious and contorts himself into a martyr's pose. The skirmishes, the bad thoughts, the laying hands on each other, and the conspiratorial silences have continued between him and my mother.

Aided by all those lies, I head out on my first date and impassively watch a movie where not even the protagonist is left alive. There's a montage of mangled bodies and decapitated heads, blood spraying like bleach, animals kicked, houses set ablaze. I don't understand if this is a test and I can't tell whether Luciano wants me to wear the dress of a sensitive small-town girl or the armor of a daughter of working-class people. Unsure, I smile at him as the credits roll and say: We should kiss.

So we do while the lights turn on. Until that moment, the only words we'd exchanged were *ciao* and *how are you*. When he reaches his hand past his seat and sticks it between my thighs, I stand up slowly and say that we'll see each other again, maybe.

In a heartbeat I'm back outside, heading toward the bus stop in front of Nero's tomb, now covered in graffiti and surrounded by beer cans. I stare at it with fondness and conviction—it's the place where, legend has it, the man who set fire to all of Rome now rests.

That Christmas, my brother decides not to show up for lunch. Grandma comes alone, taking two trains from Ostia, balancing two baking dishes with mushroom-and-prosciutto lasagna on her knees. When she arrives, she walks right in and starts critiquing everything— there's mildew near the kitchen's range hood, the grout lines aren't white, the twins make such a racket and they're so skinny, they look like breadsticks or lampposts.

We eat with the radio on. They say that people are praying with candles in hand beside the holes left at the World Trade Center. Our silence is shattered only by the twins' games, the sounds they make with their mouths, the way they snap their little fingers. They're quickly shushed and sent into a corner by my mother's glares. Meanwhile, a chill has settled over Massimo. Ever since he and Mariano were separated, they've done nothing but call each other *my son* and *my father*, which baffles Antonia and gives me the same feeling I get when I reach the epilogue of a book without having understood the ending.

Mariano's empty chair is filled with our unease. The lights strung on the balcony are the only decoration we have up, and Antonia decided that we'd spent too much this year on books, dictionaries, clothes, and toilet paper, so there won't be any gifts. After all (as she puts it) we don't lack for anything.

No one ever told the twins about Santa Claus—just as they hadn't told me or Mariano. No one hid gifts in our dressers or under our beds, and no one ever snuck into the living room at midnight to pile up gifts wrapped in shiny paper and bows.

Santa Claus is a fairy tale, and he's got nothing to do with Jesus—they invented him, Antonia always said, a theory she's proudly upheld since I was five.

At school, from the first grade on, I pretended to believe, siphoning imagination from the other kids' stories. While they endured the heartbreak of discovering that magic is nothing but a human invention, I was off constructing fantasies out of Styrofoam, fully committed to make-believe.

After lunch, I cross the street, go to the phone booth, and drop in some coins. I hear it ring and I hope Mariano picks up. I picture him at home alone, with a bag of potato chips, sitting on Grandma's wine-colored couch and staring at the windowsill or the oleander tree in the apartment building's courtyard.

Hello?

Maria', it's me.

Oh. Merry Christmas.

Merry Christmas, what are you up to?

Nothing, I was sleeping.

Why didn't you come?

Because Antonia would've flipped out, and I'm sick and tired of her.

Are you tired of me too?

No. How's Papà?

Sitting.

You're becoming as cold and hard as a rock.

And you're becoming as distant as Pluto.

Why'd you call?

I need to ask you something.

Then ask.

When boys have you touch them, do they want you to be behind them?

What kind of question is that?

Just a question. Tell me.

Behind them to do what?

To touch them—from behind. Is that how it's done or not?

No, that's not how it's done. Did someone make you do that?

No, no one. I was just curious.

The money runs out, cutting off our call and our holiday greetings. I didn't get the chance to tell him that I miss him, that without him there's nobody left who really knows me, no one who helps me carry a two-meter-tall pink bear up the stairs, no one who performs such useless yet sacred tasks with me.

I go back inside, lost in my thoughts—thoughts already far from the pandoro cake that we got 10 percent off, far from my father, who opened the bag and poured in the powdered sugar. Now he's shaking it like a maraca. It's making the dull sound of trash bags being tossed into the street.

After the movies, Luciano and I continued our courtship, exchanging glances and brushing up against each other. Our phone calls have become a regular evening ritual, but I always have to ask him to call me back, because after five minutes on the line my mother signals for me to hang up and makes the gesture of money, rubbing her fingers together—money running out, money, money, wasted money.

Our conversations float on the surface, always circling the same topics: his private English lessons, his wins and losses in soccer, if he's going to the stadium with his father, and whether I've been thinking about him. Of course, I say, a lot. I've thought about you a lot, I repeat, because I don't know how to quantify more than that.

What comes after a lot? Loads? An infinity? The entire universe? I've thought about you as much as the universe, I say, as I tear at the bits of skin around my nails.

When I'm with him, I don't touch on the difficult subject of my home life. I steer clear of existential or other uncomfortable questions. Instead, I mentally run through the list of things he has that I don't, and I almost feel like I own them, too, through our subtle, unofficial bond. I imagine that, like the principle of communicating vessels, at some point his affluence will spill over, and I'll be the one to collect it. I'm the vessel that's small and below and facing upward with an open mouth.

Samuele made sure to tell me that he and Luciano aren't friends and that Luciano isn't worth my time. He muttered his opinion to me, which I hadn't asked for, at the end of Latin class one day. I shrugged my shoulders in response.

Who cares? I said, as I carefully placed my pens back into my long, pink case.

I don't see Luciano much outside of school, though sometimes I manage to stop by the bar across the street where he spends hours chewing licorice and commenting on soccer games, those he's already played and those still to come. I just nod along, half listening. Using the excuse of going to Marta's to study, I carve out a few afternoons, and the first I spend at Luciano's house.

We take the bus together, and I can feel the other girls' eyes on me, liquid and quivering, sizing up my clothes and my backpack. They're starting to notice our closeness and struggle to understand what would make someone like Luciano want to hang out with someone like me—the soggy one, pretty but not too pretty, the girl who might have lice and whose tights are full of runs.

The villa where he lives has a laurel hedge. It's the first hedge in my life—not the first chronologically, but the first I've ever given symbolic value to—because I'd never thought about wanting one until that moment. Now, the hedge is everything I yearn for, the ability to create tall boundaries, to cordon off and exclude from sight.

Luciano's bedroom is in the basement, but one side opens onto the lower part of the yard, so it's nothing like the basements I'm used to, with their dark corners and the stale air of old buildings. Down there, in what they call the tavern, Luciano has his own bathroom and a spacious room with a pool table, like a gambling den. His room is three times the size of mine, and I discover that he collects blue Ralph Lauren sweaters—he shows them to me with great enthusiasm.

Soon we start kissing. His parents aren't home, and even if they do come back, they won't nose around and come looking for him. It's as if he lives alone, as if he were already an adult, a lawyer who could take off at any moment on a cruise across the Atlantic or to visit the North Pole.

I've never asked if he's seeing other girls, never pushed to define what we are, to draw clear lines around us. I don't know what kind of music he listens to or whether he prefers mint- or fruit-flavored gum. The only things I do know are that he has all those identical sweaters, he likes movies where the good guys get strangled alongside the bad, and he's mastered the art of combing his hair to get that perfect flip at the ends.

I can feel him making awkward attempts to rub and touch me, and I react by pulling away. I tell him that I'll be the one touching him, that I'm not interested in having his hands on me. In response he doesn't say yes, but he doesn't say no either.

But you have to turn around, I say. I don't want to look at your face.

What do you mean? he asks, and I remember: Be careful with boys—even when they tell you to trust them, even when they seem to understand, they never do.

What I mean is you should look outside. Your yard is prettier than I am.

And that's how we do it. I focus on the back of his head, and he focuses on the little yellow rosebushes outside.

How do you bring a deluge home? The others don't know, but I do.

In January, I find Antonia bent over the kitchen table, her elbows pinning down the tablecloth. She hadn't even bothered to take a seat. She's leafing through my planner, or rather, the two notebooks bound with rubber bands where she wrote down all the numbers and days of the week. She's stopped on one page, staring at it with orca eyes, huge and black.

What are these? she asks and points at the page. She presses on a square of graph paper, she presses and presses as if she wants to puncture it.

I don't know. I move closer to see what she's pointing at. She's found some of the drawings Luciano made in my planner. He stole it from me when I was at his house and, laughing, said he'd decorate it.

I hear the rain pitter-patter on the balcony, and it feels like the water is ready to invade the house, to flood the kitchen and bathroom, the beds and cabinets.

Who drew them? Antonia asks, bending over even more. She looks like a whale determined to turn me into plankton.

A friend . . .

These are Celtic, Celtic crosses—Fascist symbols—in your planner! Her voice rises ten notes, it's high-pitched, piercing. She slams the planner down on the table twice, like she's trying to turn it into confetti, and I'm on the verge of drowning. My feet are cold in wool socks; the radiators seem far away, and the temperature has dropped below zero.

Tomorrow I'm going to school with you, she shouts so loudly it feels like our balcony could collapse, taking the entire building with it. I hear the *click* of the bedroom door—my father has locked himself in.

Don't say a word. Don't even think about laughing. Don't try to run. Get over here. My mother grabs me by the elbow, opens the notebook again, and shoves my face into Luciano's drawings, as if I were a dog that peed where it shouldn't.

The next morning, she says she's not going to work. She has on her green wool hat and blue gloves—a clash of colors like the kind we once bonded over, but that I now can't stand. She escorts me on the train and all the way to school, disgust on her face, while mine shows my dismay at being unable to stop any of it.

As soon as we step into the school courtyard, I feel my mother's hand clamp around my elbow again, steering me. I keep my eyes down on the cracks in the asphalt, the holes, and the pine needles, hoping for the apocalypse to come and wipe us all out before my mother does.

Marching like a soldier, Antonia drags me to the floor where the principal's office is and posts herself in front of the door, waiting to be received. She doesn't have an appointment—she never does—but she will not budge until they open that door.

We sit down across from the principal, a small woman with short black hair. Her glasses, with their round lenses, dangle from a pearl-studded chain. Her delicate perfume smells like flowers and cardamom, and it wrestles with my mother's carpenter sweat.

Antonia opens my planner and shows it to the principal.

One of your students drew these in my daughter's notebooks.

The principal looks at it and smiles uncomfortably. She twists her fingers and tries to downplay the situation, saying that kids often see certain phrases or symbols on walls, they hear chants at the stadium, they read scribbles on the bus—it's just ignorance, just things they don't really understand, and with time, it will all be forgotten.

Dear signora, my mother says, I myself had very little schooling, and I'm not here to tell you how to teach my daughter. I won't come back here again to tell you what you should or shouldn't be doing, but I demand that she be protected. That boy needs to be called in, and his family too. These aren't just drawings.

Of course . . . I'll ask his teachers to help him understand, to talk with him—but you realize you're putting your daughter in a difficult position here . . . I know the students, and it never ends well when they start accusing one another.

I'm the one accusing him. I'm the one in a difficult position, you understand? I want an apology from that boy, from his family, and from you.

My mother stands up, the chair squeaking under her, and I stay seated, trapped in a nightmare. My hands are damp, and I can feel the two worlds I've stubbornly kept separate, in airtight compartments, beginning to blend.

They're just drawings, I want to tell her. They're just lines and circles, just pages of graph paper we can tear out. But I can't get a single syllable out of my mouth. I drown in the sterile waters of my defeat.

6

I Die a Bit in the Summer

It was May when my father broke in half—he fell from a scaffold while carrying two buckets of lime, one in each hand. Another worker tripped on a pulley and crashed into him. My father lost his balance, and the iron bar that should've protected him gave way. He let go of the buckets, but not in time to grab onto anything. When he fell, my father knew his job was off-the-books and he didn't have accident insurance and he didn't receive the usual thirteenth-month pay. Every other month he had to go ask them politely for his envelope of cash, he had to remind them of his existence, of the fact that he got up at 5:00 a.m. like everyone else to come work at the construction site. When he fell, he knew there would be no union support, there would be no protection, there would be no pressing charges.

It was May, and my father was flat on his back like a cockroach. His legs moved on their own for the last time, a spasm signaling their surrender.

A friend of his pounded on our basement door because he didn't know how to call us. The bill wasn't in our name, we didn't have a phone anymore, and of course no one on the radio mentioned my father, who had fallen, who couldn't walk, my almost-dead father. The friend knocked until my mother opened the door and then he told her: Anto', Massimo fell.

The friend had to get back to work, so my mother went out onto the street in her yellow flip-flops and the oversize T-shirt my father usually wore around the house, and she searched for someone to give us a ride. She couldn't find anyone, so she came back home, pulled on her pants, put her hair up with the usual clip, then handed one twin to each of us and said: Hold them tight, you hear me? Tight.

Mariano and I followed her, both of us small and burdened with indecision and dread. We waited at the bus stop for a bus that wasn't coming, we waited and waited while Antonia paced back and forth, acting like she didn't see us, her thoughts swirling around her like bedsheets flapping in the wind. The bus finally came and we crammed into two seats, even though there were five of us. The twins cried, then they were quiet, and then they stared up at us and cried some more. Mariano and I didn't dare ask what had happened or why; we just held our brothers tight, almost to the point of suffocating them.

By the time we were on the third bus, more than an hour had passed since we'd left home. The bus was boiling hot, the windows wouldn't open, and my mother yelled at the driver that we couldn't breathe: There's no air back here! But he didn't pull over, he didn't even check, and all the passengers in their light, summery clothes pointed and stared at us rudely.

I never want to go back to that hospital—just hearing the word *policlinico* makes me turn my face away, as if it were a crater, the scar of a cataclysm. In the emergency room, they made us sit in the waiting area, and Maicol was pressed up against my skin, making me sweat. His face looked different from mine and my mother's. I envied him because, if Papà died, Maicol still had time to look like him. Mariano, too, had figured out that whatever was happening had something to do with Massimo; he kicked the wall, holding his brother in his arms as if he were a burden.

Quit it with those feet, my mother said, and Mariano froze. Then she went and spoke with the nurses and doctors, disappearing behind a door, leaving the four of us on the edge of a cliff, ready to throw ourselves off.

People shuffled around us in slippers and nightgowns, people came out of the elevators on stretchers. Someone said, There's a code red. He fell from God knows where, probably some poor guy working in construction—and I registered those words, I registered *poor guy*, and I passed them from one synapse to another like bile on my tongue. *Poor guy.*

When Antonia came back, I noticed the sweat stains under her arms and a deep crease between her eyebrows, which hadn't looked like that earlier, it hadn't been such a furrow and valley.

She gathered us close, and touched our arms with her large hands, hands that never trembled. She didn't cry or wail, she didn't scream or curse God and the cosmos. Antonia wasn't even thirty years old, and her husband not even forty. She simply said: Papà can't walk. I need you guys to pay attention right now, okay? Are you paying attention?

Mariano and I nodded. We were in pieces. We were children. We had no toys and had no home, but we were paying attention.

We have to be strong, very, very strong, Antonia repeated. She took the twins back into her arms and sat down on a green plastic chair, surrounded by the relatives of other people who had been brought there or came in on their own two feet. She pulled out one breast at a time and nursed the twins, who sucked milk and disinfectant, milk and sickness.

Your father doesn't work in construction, are you paying attention? He doesn't work. If anyone asks, he doesn't work; he stays at home. He fell down the stairs. Now you say it.

We stayed silent, our eyes fixed on her breasts and the oversize shirt and her sweat and her red hair.

Now *you* say it, she hissed, quieter this time, and looked into our eyes—first mine, then Mariano's.

Papà doesn't work, he fell down the stairs.

Papà doesn't work, he fell down the stairs.

She nodded, satisfied with our recitation, and had us sit back down and be still.

He isn't my father, Mariano whispered in my ear, as though warding off his own anguish.

Bear says: First one who jumps off the pier wins.

But he doesn't say what.

The mopeds are parked next to the pier's steps, in the piazza where I first encountered the lake—and it's still there, the same black water, the same smell of wet feathers.

Bear isn't his real name, but it's what he likes to be called. He's two years older than me and the only person I know with a tattoo in the middle of his chest—a bear's muzzle, mouth wide-open. He says he dreamed about it when he was younger, the animal devouring him, starting from his feet, gnawing his big toe.

Marta leans with her elbows on the moped handlebars and shakes her head. She thinks jumping in is disgusting. She has straight hair and a big mole on her left nostril. School is about to end, and it looks like she'll get an A+ in conduct—perfect behavior, like she's some kind of mummy or fresco.

I start walking down the pier, my black flip-flops clapping and my body squishing from the sweat. It's already hot out, though it's only the start of the season, and the water is still cold.

The Greco takes off his shirt. He's only wearing his Bermuda swim shorts. He leaves his shoes and helmet on his moped and walks up the stairs, saying: I've done it at least ten times before.

But it's a lie. I've already figured out that everything the Greco says is a lie—his last name, the country he claims he was born in, even his father's job.

I see the Greco go past me. He has dark, almost mixed skin, and he complains that the pier is burning his feet.

I turn to face the mopeds and recognize almost everyone there: Marta, Dafne, Ramona, and Iris—none of them would even think about joining me. They don't care about winning some unknown prize.

Bear reaches the railing and shouts back at me: What, are you scared? He says it like he would to one of his guy friends.

I'm not. Are you?

I take off my T-shirt and jean shorts, leaving just my black one-piece bathing suit—the one I plan to wear all summer long, never tiring of it, loving how the spandex cools on my stomach after each swim.

Bear's eyes are glassy and red, like my brother's. He's not very tall, and he shaved his head a few months ago—Marta told me they'd had to operate on his brain. He was always in pain, and one day something must've popped inside of him, like popcorn at the movies.

He doesn't answer my question but laughs, sitting on the railing, hoping to be the first to reach the pilings we're jumping from. The Greco is right behind and tries to pass him. But from the way he hesitates, straddling the railing, I start to doubt whether he's ever jumped off before.

Be careful! Iris yells at me, taking a few steps toward us. Our eyes meet. I'm not sure whether to be flattered or confused. Her concern throws me off. Then she adds: Don't slip.

We only met recently. In fact, all of us were strangers to one another until the start of the month, when Marta invited me to spend the May 1 holiday at the lake with her cousin Bear and some other friends: the Greco, Dafne, Ramona, and Iris, who, after learning that I'd read *Pride and Prejudice*, said: I read it too.

Her response annoyed me, and for a long time I thought she was lying or trying to make fun of me. Books like that had been both a punishment and a kind of power play for me up until then. They'd excluded me from my classmates' references and conversations. I didn't watch the TV shows they watched, I didn't play the video games they played, and I didn't read the books they read.

Before the boys can make their move, I'm already standing on the railing, leaning out. I carefully place one foot, then the other, on the piling where the lake's tour boat docks. From way up here, my red hair flaps in the wind, whipping me in the face.

I feel the push starting from my ankles and I look down at the algae floating on the water's surface—they form shapes that could be mistaken for continents. I gather momentum and see the boys struggling out of the corner of my eye. Ramona shouts in dialect: Don't hurt yourself! Then I jump, and the freezing water stings my slim thighs and chin. My heels touch the lake bottom under the pier. I feel slimy rocks and dull pieces of glass. It's dark and there's nothing there—I open my eyes to see the long, blurry shadows of the algae, then push off to return to the surface. Another splash breaks the silence that had settled over me and the lake. Bear comes up for air shortly after I do.

The Greco is still sitting there on the railing, his pride tucked between his shoulder blades, the defeated face of someone who's lost a race. He's been trying to get Iris's attention for months and looks after her tenderly, but so far all he's earned are a few handshakes and reminders that they're just good friends.

You won, Bear smiles at me and does the dead man's float. He's shattered the lake's geographic shapes, his head and scar shining.

What did I win?

Nothing.

I kick my feet and legs in a disjointed rhythm, heading toward the shore like a wet dog.

I get out of the water, chilled, and walk across the rocks between pieces of trash, carefully watching where I place my feet. I'm terrified of being stabbed by a syringe—a fear Antonia instilled in me.

What are you doing still up there? Bear asks, coming out of the water and drying off. He tosses me a towel and looks back at the Greco, suspended where we'd left him.

I'm coming down now, he says, but he doesn't move.

So Bear goes back out on the pier and calmly helps him climb over the railing, getting his feet safely on the concrete, then slaps his back and says: You'll do it next time. What's the big deal?

The Greco nods with his eyes downcast, and I think about how kind Bear is, how human. I wonder: What happens when you throw a good person and a bad person into a lake together? Does the goodness get contaminated, does some of the bad wash away? Does it all blend together?

I stand barefoot on the dark asphalt, and after a bit, I decide to go retrieve my flip-flops and the clothes I left at the end of the pier.

You didn't even think about it, you just threw yourself in, Iris says from behind me, her black, layered hair blowing in the wind along with her little yellow checkered dress with bows on the straps.

Somebody's gotta do it.

Do what?

Throw themselves in.

She smiles and waits for me in the middle of the pier.

Do you want to come over and meet my dwarf rabbit? His name is Laurie, like, you know . . .

You should've named him Darcy—Laurie is just the guy Jo said she wouldn't be caught dead marrying, I say, showing off knowledge that now feels justified, like there's finally a place for it.

The moped engines start up. I towel dry my hair and put on the helmet Bear offers me, a loose-fitting bowl covered with colorful stickers.

Iris does the same, climbing on behind the Greco.

I know how to make pastry cream, she yells out to me, laughing despite my unfriendly response, while the mopeds take off with the loud *vroom* of their modified mufflers.

THE BITTER WATER OF THE LAKE · 127

I think about how the two things have nothing in common, absolutely nothing—pastry cream and rabbits.

Luciano is my jewel, my gold nugget, my treasure chest boyfriend, my precious adornment, the brooch of shimmering stones that I wear on my jacket lapel.

My mother hates hearing his name; she twists her lips as if struck by a whip every time he comes up. To fix the mess with the Celtic drawings, I had to tell Luciano that the problem was my mother.

You know, Lucia', my mother has all these fixations. She grew up like a crooked branch. She suffers from severe persecutory delusions: she can't tell what's right from what's wrong. She dresses like a man and pays the bills—just have pity on her, try to understand. All you need to do is apologize and then this will all be over.

Once I decided that the problem wasn't Luciano's drawings but Antonia herself, I put on a red blouse and a shiny headband Agata had given me for Christmas. I sat on the wall with my arms crossed, wearing a grave expression like someone facing the flames of an armed conflict. I looked him straight in the eye and touched my temple with my pointer finger, twisting it back and forth as though winding up a music box, to signal that all my mother's phobias lived upstairs, in her head.

After Luciano's apology, I was banned from talking to him—a ban I methodically broke by using my friends' cell phones at school and sneaking into the hallways behind the auditorium to see him. I gave him letters written on the backs of graph paper full of math problems. I drew hearts for him, angels with small, asymmetrical wings, and wrote phrases of a synthetic, plexiglass kind of love. The more you say it—*I love you*—the more it disintegrates, like wax that drips and runs, getting all over the floor.

School's out for the year and I maintained my A- average. My mother saw my report card and said they could've made an effort to give me an A, so I pointed out my A in Italian. Seeing it, she tried to keep a straight face, suppressing her satisfaction beneath her quivering lips.

For the last conference before our report cards, my Italian teacher had wanted to meet with my parents. Only Antonia showed up, and the teacher handed her a writing exam booklet with my composition in it. She told her she gave me an A+ but that she was worried because I'd written about a fountain filled with fish in an apartment building's courtyard, about how my hand moved in circles while my mouth stayed shut, and how people yelled down at me from their windows: Shame on you! I had written about how, with my tiny fingers, I squeezed the fish one by one and made their eyes pop out of their smooth bodies, pulled their tails, and scraped off their scales. The teacher told my mother that the composition was well written— I had a better vocabulary than every other student in the class—but something was tormenting me.

Back at home, my mother wasted no time in asking: Is something tormenting you? You have to tell me.

No, nothing.

I defended myself by snatching the composition from her hands. In it, I had condemned my younger self—my helpless childhood and innocent games, when I didn't know how to fight and I'd wait for Antonia to defend me, when I'd run to her or Mariano and tell them about the attacks I'd endured.

But maybe I should've screamed: It's you! You're clearly the one tormenting me, along with the rest of the world, and all the things I don't have—a TV, for starters, the shows on Italia 1, blonde highlights, soccer-player figurines, a Game Boy, a PlayStation, *Tomb Raider*, all the books you won't let me read, bright Lelli Kelly shoes, Chupa Chups to suck on every afternoon without having you say my teeth will fall out, puffs of a cigarette without being afraid of ending up on some park bench, swim class, volleyball, theater, a cell phone that rings and rings and never stops, birthday parties at McDonald's, a Guess purse to match the shoes, endless pairs of Nike and Adidas sneakers, Sundek swimsuits, Winnie the Pooh T-shirts, Festivalbar compilations, Britney Spears CDs, afternoons at underage discotecas, a minicar, a moped with neon lights under the pedals, Big Babol gum to chew in class, hashish to melt in my palm, and my brother's glassy, red eyes . . . Everything tormented me. Everything. Including the fish that remained silent, even while people were accusing me.

This is why an A in Italian feels to us like an insult: My daughter is a good writer, but she writes about malice. She wastes beautiful words on cruel things.

School ends and Luciano leaves for Sardinia with his family. They have a house on the coast and a boat—he doesn't think to invite me. I haven't received a single gift from him since we started dating. He doesn't want to share his luxurious life with me. He keeps me confined between the walls of our school and in outings nearby. I'm good enough to be naked in his room, but not to fraternize with his friends.

At our class dinner, to say goodbye at the end of the school year, I order a pizza margherita because it's the cheapest thing on the menu. I drink sparkling water, and I'm wearing that headband that makes me look like a catechist, and a big sweatshirt that makes me look like a basketball player. Samuele shows up at some point with his two buddies. He's been drinking and he staggers toward the table, starts clapping in front of our teachers, and bows, swaying, in the middle of the room. He thanks them for flunking him again.

Everyone freezes, as though posing for a painting, hands resting on the paper tablecloth, legs crossed under the table—our teachers sit like statues made of plaster, trapped by their meager salaries and arrogant colleagues.

I stand up and walk around the table, take Samuele by the arm, and guide him toward the door. He lets himself be led, muttering under his breath.

Go home now, I tell him, releasing him outside the restaurant. I look at his friends. They're the same ones from the roof. You didn't study anything all year, and now you come here and cause a scene? Samuele's face is pale, his forehead sweaty. Something is gurgling on his lips.

What do you have inside you, rocks? he asks, then doubles over and vomits right in front of me, at the edge of a manhole. I watch as the rivulets of his gastric juices snake across the asphalt, remnants of a fast-food dinner.

I turn around and head back inside—I won't have my evening ruined. I got the grades I deserved, I have a rich boyfriend, and I have an entire summer ahead of me. For people my age, summer is like mass, like church. It's like reaching a riverbank after a long swim, breathing fresh air after a stifling car ride, or an entire town dressing up for a party.

I sit back down next to Agata.

What happened? she asks, nervously.

He threw up, I say, cutting a slice of my now-cold pizza.

He scares me, but I also feel a bit sorry for him, she whispers.

My pizza's cold, I grumble, chewing on rock-hard mozzarella. *Clink clink*. I loudly toss my utensils onto the plate.

His name is Batman.

Who?

My rabbit.

I thought you said it was Laurie.

His name changed. He didn't even notice.

Behind Iris's house, there's a small vegetable garden marked off by petrol-green netting, with lettuce, tomatoes, cabbage, broccoli, and a rabbit named Batman. He's black and fights crime, squashing any snails that dare attack the kale.

Iris is the first person I've met in Anguillara with a house like mine. We live two kilometers away from each other, and even though her family isn't in public housing, their apartment is like ours: kitchen, bathroom, two bedrooms, one living room.

Our flip-flops are caked with dirt and Iris is searching for Batman among the bamboo canes her grandpa uses for the San Marzano tomatoes to climb.

There used to be a parrot named Crest in there, she says, pointing at a tall, empty cage.

I don't ask what happened to the bird. Instead, I steal an unripe strawberry and suck its acidity down into my belly.

Every day, I have to come up with a new way to reach the lake. Recently, the son of the family my mother works for gave up his bicycle, so I inherited it. I'm learning to ride it in front of the house—I've already fallen twice and my knees are scraped up like a child's. I can't rely on it for transport yet, so I have to take the town's shuttle bus to the lakeshore or walk to Iris's house, where, hidden from our parents, Bear and the Greco come get us on their mopeds (even though doubling up like that is illegal). Or sometimes Marta's grandma swings by in her bell-pepper-yellow Fiat Punto and gives us a ride.

Iris shares a room with her sister, and their walls are decorated with childhood photos, as well as some blue-and-white Lazio soccer pennants, their family's beloved team. She showed me her bookshelf, timidly, because she doesn't own many books. Most of what she reads come from the library, but she's still eager to list off what she's read. She has a notebook where she writes down all the books she's ever read and whether she liked each one. She hasn't shown it to me yet, but it made me feel a strong urge to make up for it. I don't keep a list like that and I've never thought to make one. I've already forgotten many of the novels I've read, and there are millions I've yet to read.

I imagine the unread books lined up like a firing squad—sooner or later, they'll shoot me.

Ever since Agata left for a few months of language study in England—thanks to her failing grade in English at the end of the year—Iris has become my daily friend. I still refuse to ask about Carlotta. Whenever someone brings her up, I say with dramatic flair: Carlotta who?

From June on, Iris and I fall into the same routine every day: we meet around 10:00 a.m., head to the lake until 5:00 p.m., then go home for dinner. For both of us, it's forbidden to disappear for the whole day. On weekends, we're allowed out until 10:00 p.m. at the latest, because after that, Antonia calls the police. It's not a joke; she actually does it. Her cop friend will come find me, asking around: Where's Antonia the Redhead's daughter? before driving me home.

Iris hands me Batman. His ears are fleshy and there's a splash of white on his nose. His black fur shines and his sharp teeth look ready for a meal.

He doesn't bite, Iris assures me, reading my mind.

I run my fingers along his smooth coat, dark like a night watchman's uniform. His yellow eyes look like lemons tossed in a bowl.

After fifteen minutes, we hear the horns of the boys' mopeds and grab our backpacks—stuffed with towels, sunscreen, and books. For weeks now, I've been pretending to like Dostoevsky's *The Idiot* and Iris has been eagerly flipping through Jack London's *Martin Eden*, constantly sighing and asking me for help with the more complicated words. I haven't told her about my dictionary—I'm still reading it and I've started underlining words since it's the only book I own and it doesn't have to be returned. I've even circled some words in red ink: *coward, moonless, anthropomorphism*. Somehow she must've caught on that I have a way with words.

June passes by: towels spread out on a hard, black beach; climbing onto each other's shoulders and diving into the water headfirst; eating Algida gelato at a summer bar; sitting in dark plastic chairs under Coca-Cola-branded umbrellas. My blotchy sunburn makes me look like a calf, and my father's huge sunglasses slide off my nose whenever I sneeze. I never put my red hair up, not even when my neck is sweaty, because I can't reveal my elephant ears. My freckles are out of control, dotting my arms and legs. Sometimes Bear takes a pen from the bar and connects them, tracing constellations on my skin: bats, starfish, windmills.

My favorite pastime is chicken fighting. When we're not playing Smash Seven with the Super Tele ball or doing handstands and flips, I get Iris to climb up on my shoulders, and together we challenge nearby contenders. In this way, our strength and our moves are doubled, while our desire for war and victory quadruples.

Whenever there's an underwater-breath-holding competition, I'm in. I cross my legs, close my eyes, and force all the air out of my lungs until I find myself sitting on the lake bed. Then I begin to count. I train myself to never surrender. I move my hands to stay down there and not resurface, until my head starts spinning.

Iris doesn't like seeing me go under for too long. She usually stands nearby and scans the water above my head. When she no longer sees any bubbles, she starts swirling her fingers, making little whirlpools underwater to warn me she's about to intervene. Then she grabs me by the hair—like a cat with its newborns—and pulls me back into the world.

For lunch, we eat hot dogs with melted cheese singles, tuna-and-tomato sandwiches, or, in Iris's case, white bread and mayo. Then we find a shady corner to read in and swap deeds and misdeeds from our novels. These conversations with her make all the hours spent in front of the page worthwhile—some pages I like, some I hate, and some deserve to be torn out and used as parchment paper.

I've already expressed my loathing of Prince Myshkin to Iris multiple times. He drives me crazy with his pure ways and his white phlegm. If he were in front of me, I'd slap him.

I hate innocent people, I say, and Iris starts laughing.

Dafne told us that her mom doesn't let her read books like ours because she says they aren't educational and we're still too naive for them at our age. She prefers making her daughter memorize Bible verses and spend her days cleaning beaches or forests with the Girl Scouts. That's how I learned that there are worse parents in the world than mine.

One Saturday night, bored and tired, we find ourselves in the Piazza del Molo, as usual. Bear disappears with the Greco on a moped, leaving us girls sitting on the wall, people watching, deciding who to greet and who to ignore, remarking on everyone's pasts and possible futures. Iris is great at doing imitations and giving nicknames, so in our secret language of gestures and sounds, we're able to gossip about people's predicaments and private lives without them ever knowing.

It's almost 10:00 p.m., my curfew is approaching, and the boys still haven't returned. I pace back and forth with my arms folded across my chest like a cruel legion commander.

Finally, we see them driving into the piazza in an old car. It reeks and only one headlight works. They stole it from the Greco's neighbor and are driving it without a license and without seat belts on, their beardless faces smug. They turn sharply and the tires squeal, then they come to a stop right in front of us. Bear rolls down the windows and cranks up the volume on the old stereo, tuned to Radio Vaticana—broadcasting prayers and penance, even on a Saturday night. The word of Christ rings out into the piazza, drowning out the shouts and laughter around us.

Bear climbs onto the hood and stands up to bless the crowd, arms wide, full of goodness and wisdom. He cries out to the few onlookers: You will never be free of me.

Radio Vaticana is our town's faithful companion, not because the townsfolk are particularly pious, but because the radio's repeaters are just a few kilometers from our houses. With their waves, the radio can somehow be heard whenever we respond to our intercoms, our landlines, even when we open our refrigerator doors. There, thanks to the artificial light illuminating the food, we're inundated by divine will and, together with the salami and lettuce, we contemplate the kingdom of heaven.

Iris and I are overcome with laughter though I'm not one to laugh easily. My stomach hurts from the hilarity of the scene: the ugly car, the rotten stench coming from the muffler, Bear looking like some saintly figure, house music replaced by the family rosary.

The Greco convinces us to go for a spin. We roll down the windows, stick our arms out, sing "Almeno tu nell'universo," recite insults, curse words, and blasphemies—all while Radio Vaticana wishes the faithful a good night. Dafne's face is red, she says her head hurts. The car sputters along, stalling because the Greco doesn't actually know how to drive.

We laugh about our omnipotence.

The roads outside town are dark and we race past a pizzeria. I tell Bear to slow down, but he takes the next curve with determination. The lake's water glints—it's the blade of a knife, slicing the houses in two.

I'm wearing black plastic heels that are shiny and killing my feet. The sticker-covered helmet wobbles on my head. This is my first pair of heels. They have straps around the ankles and the clasps bite into my skin.

It's my debut night, my grand entrance into society. I'm all dressed up for the discoteca. I told my mother I was going to a harmless pajama party at Marta's. It took some time for her to come around because she's uneasy about my new friends, who she knows so little about. My father, on the other hand, said to her: If it were Mariano . . .

We pass the sailing club and keep straight. The moped's engine has been modified—it's going faster than it should. Yesterday, a squad car stopped us on the wrong side of the road—I wasn't wearing a helmet, Bear was grinning. The cop recognized me and said: It's only because of your mother that I'm not taking you to the station. I wanted to maul him.

Bear doesn't use his signal, he just turns between the houses, and at the end of the road I see it—that coal-black tongue, smelling of slimy algae and dense sand: the lake.

We take the road that runs alongside it, spreading our legs wide as a wave of mugginess hits us. The beach clubs are closed, and the newspaper stand has its usual two inflatable toys dangling by their necks—a yellow dinosaur and a speckled turtle. I call them the Hanged Ones.

Bear zigzags between backed-up cars. It's a one-way road, and the lakefront bars are filling up. Parking spots are running low. He plants his feet on the ground and grumbles. We're stuck between a red car and a giant flowerpot. I can already see the beams of light swirling in the sky above the discoteca. The people walking past us must've parked long before the turn off the main road.

We've lost the others, I tell Bear, and pinch the skin his helmet doesn't cover. He yelps.

The smell of horses wafts from the stables one street over. The sand is always moist and the asphalt warm. Only two years ago, the discoteca we're heading to was just a shaved-ice shack. Now it has an enormous Japanese pagoda in the middle, lacquered and glossy. I've only ever seen it during the day, and I've dreamed of its bewitching presence, its seductive power. There must be wizards and fairies inside.

We finally manage to get through and park on the gravel on the side of the road. There's a line to get into the club.

Everyone's wearing dress shirts, I point out to Bear.

He smooths down his plain white T-shirt and gets in line. We spot Marta with Ramona. Dafne had to stay home—her mom didn't fall for the story of a pajama party with supposedly studious schoolgirls.

I don't need a dress shirt, Bear says and makes his way through the crowd, greeting everyone he knows, shaking hands. His charm melts their reticence, making him seem older, like a thirty-year-old in a pinstripe suit.

We cling to him. Girls get in free, and we pretend we're at least seventeen. We're young, fresh prey, and our hearts are in our throats. The curtain separating us from the club is a threshold—beyond it, anything can happen. We'll turn into Amazons, warriors, and princesses.

Once inside, we find Iris almost immediately. She's holding a tall plastic cup in her hands (the kind they give you in the VIP section), wearing a white blouse with a tie at the neck and sandals with fake jewels around the ankles, and her hair has been freshly dyed by her mother's hairdresser.

I walk over and see that the bow on her blouse has come undone, exposing her bra. I step closer and quickly retie it. She smiles, though the alcohol has muted it, and says: Thank you.

Hand, bow, smile. Thank you.

It's crowded. We squeeze through to get to the bar, which is red and black, decorated with gold dragons. I feel nauseated and order a mojito, something I've never tried before, but it doesn't feel right to just ask for a soda. I suck the cane sugar up from the bottom with a straw. The lime has an acrid smell, and Iris says something I can't hear. We're overlooking an artificial pond that three red carp have been dumped into.

I try to not lose the others, I follow their backs with my eyes. I spot Bear chatting with the Greco and some of their friends. Marta and Ramona stand like lonely, abandoned lampposts on a country road, lost in the din of a place that isn't meant for us.

Then someone touches my back, and I turn to find Andrea lurking behind me like a crow or an owl. My head starts throbbing, like when I'm running a fever or have been in the sun too long. His face is clean and pleasant, as usual, his eyes are bright, and he's wearing a buttoned-up burgundy dress shirt. He asks me who I'm here with and why, then says: Somebody threw a rock at my dad's windshield. Do you have any idea who it was?

His cologne smells like wood and almonds. His eyes flit around above my head, unable to focus, like he's looking for something beyond me. Iris watches him, perplexed, and snaps: That has nothing to do with us. We have to go, and she grabs my wrist and tries to pull me away.

Andrea acts as if Iris were simply a shadow and ignores her, then everything happens very quickly. I move toward Iris. Andrea keeps looking around and then smirks, as if he's just seen a rat galloping past. Someone says: Whatcha lookin' at?

I turn to see a boy with large ears, a crew cut shaved close at the temples, small close-set eyes, and an untucked light-blue dress shirt with a rigid collar. He's got a tattoo on his wrist and walks with his legs wide, as if he were riding a horse, or a tractor.

Whatcha lookin' at? he repeats, and Andrea replies, without a trace of dialect, that he's not looking at anything.

I stare at the boy's face, trying and failing to recall his name. The boy's gaze is blank—he shoves Andrea without warning. Iris and I are like glass crystals, the light of what's about to happen passing right through us.

Andrea says: Were you the one who threw the rock?

The boy says no and starts to laugh.

Then why are you laughing? Andrea takes a step closer and the boy shoves him again.

Iris mutters a *Cut it out*, but no one listens. People are staring. They seem to be expecting a show, like the fireworks at the fish festival.

I approach the boy and touch his elbow lightly, saying: Give it a rest.

He looks me over and says: I know who you are.

Suddenly, we're outside the club. Iris stayed behind and said she'd go find Bear and the Greco. Andrea and the boy have declared battle and, as everyone knows, when you fight you have to pick a place, you have to make a date to draw your swords. If they had gauntlets, they would've thrown them down by now.

I couldn't help but follow them. I'm always drawn to trouble, to commotion, to brawls. My first night as a debutante is already winding down, the script weak, the strobe lights flickering in the distance, and the mojito churning in my stomach.

The two are still at it, threatening each other, and the boy's dialect is growing thicker. He hurls insults I've never heard before. They keep shoving each other, and soon Andrea is almost at the water's edge, the boy is driving him toward the water.

I scream: Enough!

Andrea looks at me with the distant eyes of an astronaut. You can hear the lake lapping against the shore and a calm breeze ripples the surface. You can almost see the patina of sunscreen on the water, a remnant from the day that will keep the fish from ever swimming close to shore.

Cristia', I know it was you, Andrea accuses him again.

The boy, Cristiano, has red cheeks and his shirt is half unbuttoned. He looks like he's been drinking, like someone who hears the thunderous world crashing in his head. Take a hike, he orders Andrea, who lunges again, so I put myself between them.

No one cares about your windshield, idiot, I yell at Andrea and push him away.

Cristiano smiles as if this were the beginning of something, a window opening onto a beautiful view.

Carlotta stares at her bed—she's had the same sheets since childhood—then takes out a transparent bag, made for packaging bread, for a loaf that's at least one kilogram.

She has a modular bedroom, a full-size bed, a bridge wardrobe, a matching soap-pink desk, and on top of it are her schoolbooks, a roll of tape, and some scissors—the scissors are there in case she changes her mind.

Carlotta opens her wardrobe and looks at her outfits. There are so many, but she can only choose one. She runs her fingers from the green velvet dress (unsuitable for the season) to the one with the bold flower print (too exuberant for the occasion). Way in the back, she touches the dress from her communion with her fingertips. It's ruffled and white, like something a child bride would wear.

In the end, she decides to remain as she is: wearing a pair of black leggings that accentuate her hips, a loose T-shirt with the Superman *S* on it. She takes off her socks. She has red polish on her toenails and feels like the color goes well with everything, with what's about to happen.

She sits on the bed, looks over at the socks she's thrown into a corner, and picks up her cell phone to reread the last texts she's received. They're all from the same sender, they all say the same words. She doesn't have the number saved because she doesn't know who is texting her.

Her eyes are dilated and her eyelids are swollen. It's as if she were seeing double: two tables, two shelves, two rolls of tape, two Carlottas. One of them is sitting on the bed and the other is scrutinizing her, standing next to the window. The second Carlotta judges her—she hates her hair, her breasts, her genitals, her skin.

Her head is full of gaps and rifts, knots and tangles. The pills she stole from her mother are beginning to take effect. She feels light, small, and impalpable. The outlines of things appear blurry. She leans out and grabs the tape with her hands. Time moves backward, folding in on itself, just like her memory, which can't recall the beginning, the exact moment she arrived, the moment she set foot in the world.

She suspects the bag has a hole in it and she checks it, turning it over in her hands. She blows into it like it's a balloon and shakes it. She obsessively traces its edges with her nails.

She finds no leaks or escape routes, so she proceeds.

It's July. The radio says that the Senate of the Republic has approved the Bossi-Fini immigration law and the return of the Savoy family to Italy. Carlotta Sperati is in her room—she's not even fifteen years old. She pulls the bag over her head and secures it around her neck with the tape, wrapping it around and around until every leak is closed off. The bag swells and deflates with her breathing. The scissors are still on the desk. Her eyes are open, and all she sees is a white ceiling and the blades of the fan spinning. She thinks about how wrong the past is—it should be shredded with a fork and knife, like Sunday roast.

Or at least, this is how I would've written her ending in a story titled: "I Die a Bit in the Summer."

7

This House Is a Disaster

The bluish light made Carlotta's eyes look enchanted, the colors on the screen reflecting in her irises. She moved the mouse and hovered the arrow over a folder named LOVE, clicked twice, and opened it for us to see.

I sat only a handspan away; it was hot, the window was ajar, and we could hear her dog dragging something around the courtyard, maybe a piece of iron. It made a *clang clang* sound whenever it crashed into anything.

For me, computers were like something out of a sci-fi movie. I belonged to the Paleolithic era of technology, the age of toasters, washing machines, radio frequencies—what was normal for others felt like the future for me.

I peered at the desktop as though it was a treasure map. When the folder opened, digital photos appeared. They were of men, naked, each photo saved with a name and a city: Alberto from Bari, Francesco from Pisa, Giuseppe from Montefiascone. There were a lot—maybe fifty—I didn't count.

In my family, we don't have any reverence for photographs. We saved only a handful from when Mariano and I were little, taken by my father with his Canon, most of which were out of focus or blurry. In some, my father's thumb made an appearance; in others, Antonia had her mouth wide-open, her eyes closed. Many were taken with the flash on sunny days, leaving us with red or overly bright eye sockets, looking like aliens or bats. They were stuffed into a few albums with black covers, inherited from my paternal grandmother, who I'd never met. After my father's accident, there were no more photos. We had nothing left to remember. Maybe my father had given his Canon to another family that needed to create memories, not bury them.

Agata asked: And what do you do? Do you send them yours?

Carlotta nodded: Of course.

She opened MSN and showed us her contacts—mostly men— and the conversations they had late into the night, the photos they attached, their declarations of mutual attraction, of pleasure and pride in their exposed, shared bodies.

As Carlotta described each of their traits, I began to feel dizzy. My temples throbbed with disgust. I don't know if it was panic, fear, or just discomfort, but I had to stand up and look at all that nudity from above. It felt aggressive, like it was sticking to the skin of my arms.

I realized, standing there in Carlotta's room, next to her computer and near the bookshelf where she still kept her stuffed bears and bunnies neatly arranged, that there was another difference between us: While she sprinted ahead and threw herself into life, I plodded behind, always at risk of falling.

The idea that someone could save a naked photo of me was horrifying. Simply the thought of it—the uncertainty, the possibility—tightened my throat and sent icy chills from the back of my neck down my legs. I'd never exposed myself in that way. I'd never undressed in front of anyone who wasn't a close friend or family member, and I couldn't imagine ever doing so. The thought that one day some Sergio from Caltanissetta would ask for a photo of me, and that I'd offer one, saying: Here, do you like it? My breasts are small, but I'm the right kind of thin—not bony, not fat. I'm a top-quality cut of meat—it seemed impossible.

Two or three chats lit up on her screen as I was having these thoughts, and Carlotta led us down the rabbit holes of her late-night conversations. She sent kisses and hugs, smileys, hearts—so many hearts—and flirted playfully. She asked them what they were doing, where they were sitting, and she laughed.

I envied her ease with others, what at the time seemed to me like a contagious and absolute sense of freedom. Her body, whether posed in front of a bathroom mirror or sitting on the bed, seemed to represent virtue and ability.

Agata seemed impressed too. She pointed at different boys and asked for more details. She even took part in the chats, trying her hand at responding, tapping on the keys at the cadence of a sleepwalker—like someone who gets out of bed at night, following a voice, and wanders out into the street.

I didn't know how to participate or what to share. I felt damaged, injured by my inability to join in—by my unspoken but obvious, boundless modesty.

I still couldn't figure out why exactly I was so modest. I didn't question where it came from—whether it stemmed from the ghostly distance that had grown over the years between my parents, whether it was a temporary, permanent, or terminal condition. I didn't know if I would ever be able to free myself from myself, or if I had somehow absorbed the ghost of past judgments, of others' gazes and opinions. I only knew that I didn't belong there. I didn't belong to that computer, those assertions of presence, or that unbearable, suffocating night.

Send me photos, one of the sleepwalkers wrote, and Carlotta didn't reply. She told us she'd send them the next day. She didn't like this guy much anyway. He had very little hair on his head and ugly hands. He was forty years old.

I was still standing and my friends hadn't taken their eyes off the computer. No one had noticed my discomfort. I was alone but safe, my weaknesses completely ignored.

I moved to the bed, and it wasn't long before Carlotta and Agata followed, lying down next to me. We didn't even cover ourselves with the sheet. The computer was still on, casting a cone of light across our faces, and I felt like I was being watched in my pajama shorts, with my bad haircut. I saw the shadow of my ears reflected and imagined it traveling through the ether, reaching all the other continents.

How about we each share a secret? Carlotta proposed from her place in the middle. We were at her sides like faithful handmaidens, adorning her bed.

I'll start, Agata said. I hate my father, I hate pigs and cows and our farm, I can't stand seeing my last name on a sign that says SAUCE TOMATOES FOR SALE. It's awful.

Carlotta said something in response and they exchanged opinions while I wondered whether, on the rare occasions when I'd bought clothes in a store, anyone in the changing rooms had ever secretly taken a photo of me in my underwear. If they had, where was I now? In which folder on their precious computer was I saved? Did I have a name? Did I have a number? Was there a specific time of day when they opened me on their desktop and examined me?

What's yours? Carlotta asked me. She had just finished telling us her secret and I hadn't been listening.

I stayed silent. It wasn't like me to take part in this kind of conversation. Usually, I was a great listener or a passive extra in their discussions, but this was my moment to speak up. I had plenty to serve on a silver platter: from my father's accident to the neighborhood I used to live in; from my brother's political beliefs to the way Antonia shaved her legs in the bidet without closing the door—but that's not what they wanted to hear. They weren't waiting for a list of my family quibbles. They wanted something personal, something from one of my darkest recesses—a real confession.

Carlotta's eyes were waiting for me to leap into the void, to surrender myself as a seal of our friendship, and I realized that my secret was this: if the two of them were to disappear, if I were to count to three and see them vanish, I probably wouldn't miss a single thing about them.

Perhaps I would have despaired about returning to the solitude that had been my closest companion since childhood, or perhaps I would have felt that I had lost a role—that I would no longer be able to call myself a good friend. Who knows what I would've done in the afternoons, where I would've gone, or what I would've been for other people.

I'm afraid of suspension bridges, I said instead. I couldn't even walk across them at the playground when I was a child.

Agata and Carlotta seemed mildly satisfied. One of them gave me a reassuring smile as if to tell me it's not that serious, I'd survive. After all, there was only one bridge in town, and no one had ever expected me to jump off it.

Thank you for your secrets, Carlotta said, closing her eyes. I kept mine glued to the screen, and that's when I noticed a small, round object perched on top of the computer. It looked like a dark eye, a giant pupil, a camera lens pointed like a gun.

What is that thing? I asked, forgetting what we had just been talking about.

A webcam, Agata said, smiling at my foolish question. It's for video calls. This way you can see the other person without having to leave the house.

I nodded and reached for an edge of the sheet to cover myself with.

The dog, meanwhile, hadn't let go of whatever he'd found, and its *clang clang* resounded in the courtyard and out along the country road.

Inviting someone over to my house would mean exposing them to my family. There's no hope of ever finding it empty. Even at sunrise, even when it's time for school or work, my father is always there.

Antonia calls him our legless watchman. He certainly won't be able to fend off thieves, but he will be witness to their theft, a marble presence.

The truth is that there's nothing to steal in our home. If there's money in the drawers or under the beds, I never knew about it. I'm sure my mother keeps it well hidden, probably in her underwear or tucked between her breasts. I wouldn't be surprised if she were to go so far as to swallow it before letting it get taken away.

What would a thief make of the shoeboxes Antonia uses to keep socks separate from shirts in our drawers; the egg cartons she paints blue, silver, and violet and keeps on a shelf in her room, filling them with trinkets, rings, and little necklaces she made with shells from Ostia and parcel twine; or the trivets made out of corks from the red and sparkling wines my father loves, but that make my temples ache?

Perhaps the unwanted guest would think we're a very creative family, that we all sit around the kitchen table with paintbrushes and markers, devoting ourselves to whimsical works of bricolage and decoupage. But that's not the reality. Decoupage is one of Antonia's favorite Sunday activities; she cuts napkins into flowers and uses PVA to glue them onto random wood surfaces (bedside tables, dressers, broom handles). The house and its ornamentation, the organizational system and its decoration, are all Antonia's doing. They are her offshoots, her creations.

Life imposes a reuse and zero-waste regime on us, and all life passes through my mother. She's the cook of stale bread, of meatballs with peas from the previous evening, of the rice omelet. She likes to flatten our leftovers in a bowl with a fork, throw eggs on top, and bake it all in the oven, regardless of the combination of spices or flavors—ours is not a cuisine for discerning palates, but for survival. Antonia learned from her mother and grandmother to not let even one drop of coffee go to waste; to fry the peels of potatoes, apples, and pears; to assemble soups with everything from vegetables to boiled meat, from the pasta left at the bottom of the box to the herbs she's dried in upside-down bunches out on the balcony.

I wonder how the thief, if invited as a guest to our dinner table, might react to our weekly obsessions: meat on Mondays—one hamburger each; gnocchi on Thursdays—which Antonia and I make, though often the gnocchi is too big and resembles whole potatoes; and fish Fridays—usually off-brand fish sticks or cod rolled in breadcrumbs and pan-fried, a symbol of our family's unity.

My father is one of those people who, despite years of eating the same meals cooked the same way by the same person, always finds something to comment on—some detail that irks him, like the amount of salt or the onions, the Parmesan or the too-thin cuts of meat. He grumbles as though trying to escape the monotony of our meals.

When I go to lunch at my friends' houses, I often see them leaving food on their plates. I hear them complain about the consistency of the pasta or the toughness of the chicken, express preferences about what's being served. At my house, I have no say over the food. Instead, I always have to show my approval of the menu, keep the twins from getting up while we eat, defend our food against Massimo's grievances. The most proven method is coughing; I cough whenever he speaks.

For as long as Mariano lived with us, breakfast, lunch, and dinner were open battlefields. He was picky about grilled vegetables, and he'd tense up over the color of the wine, over the amount of vinegar in the salad. But now that Mariano is gone, Massimo's timid efforts are quickly suppressed.

A visitor to our home would also notice the unfair disparity between my bedroom—quite large, with enough space for a huge pink bear—and the small room for the twins, who are now eight years old. So far, no one has suggested we swap, but I sense the day approaching when they'll be old enough to demand it, to have strong opinions, to claim my place.

The only relationship between me, Maicol, and Roberto is one of habit. The age gap separating us feels unbridgeable. They belong to a different geological era and speak a language I don't recognize. I'm not at all interested in how they're starting to no longer look like each other, in how their tastes are becoming more apparent, in the curlier hair of one or the thicker hair of the other, in how they say *Mamma* and *Ma'*, in how they obey while remaining calm and composed.

Unlike me and Mariano, their relationship with my mother is one of total subservience and no anger. They spend most of their time with her and even seem happy about it, still clinging to her as if they wished to undress her and drain her milk, her thoughts.

When my mother takes Massimo's sweatpants off and sits with him on the bed to massage his legs with a lotion she made, while she lifts and lowers his thighs and moves his kneecaps around and touches his hips and his bones, which seem to be getting shorter with every passing year, the twins also sit on the bed and observe the ritual up close. They learn how it should be done, conscious of the inconvenient legacy we will inherit: Papà will never walk again, and if it's not Antonia, we'll be the ones who have to invent an ointment for him, a salve to prevent his decay.

I observe those intimate, surreal moments from a distance, like a thief behind a ski mask—outcast and unknown.

It's been over a year since Mariano has shared this messy mix of emotions with me. Without him, I'm an only child and the only child who feels like a burden in her own home.

The day Iris asks if she can come over and see my room, I tell her no, because my room is small, dirty, and there's nothing to see, not even books, since I borrow and return all of them. But she insists that she doesn't care what it's like, she just wants to see where I sleep. I've seen where she sleeps.

Our reciprocity scares me. The thought of her eyes on everything I consider unmentionable bothers me.

And yet she eventually comes to my building and up the stairs to my apartment, walks through the door, sees my father in his chair next to the silent radio, and says: Buongiorno. He responds with a curt buongiorno, but she doesn't notice. She doesn't ask any questions, doesn't focus on our oddities, on our strangeness. She just follows me to my room and sits on the ground with her back up against the giant bear. She says I have a beautiful home—that's what she said—she really likes it, it's colorful and lively. She can't stand her mother's obsession with parquet floors and maintaining an immaculate living room. Our houses are the same size, but lifeblood flows in mine.

Where did you find this? she asks, resting her head against the bear.

I won it, shooting at the carnival, I confess, sitting on my bed, looking around for something to put away, for anything that appears out of place or garish.

That's so you.

What?

Shooting and winning.

Why?

Because that's just how you are. You have the courage to do anything.

I don't know what to say. I've never thought of myself as capable or strong-willed. I've only ever acted on instinct, out of feelings of revenge and shame.

One detail comes to mind from when I came across this definition: courage, noun [from Old Occitan *coratge*, Old Fr. *corage*, from Vulgar Lat. *coratĭcum*, derived from Lat. *cor*, Ital. *cuore*, "heart"].

Courage has to do with the heart, with how much heart you put into something and how far you go with it, with the blood that pumps, the arteries, the veins, the beats, the flow, the movement of the soul, the pressure, and the surge of willpower. Personally, I don't like hearts. I don't like drawing them, miming them with my fingers, coloring them in the margins, seeing them all over the stationery store in February, finding them printed on fabrics and slippers. I only use hearts—pink, red—when I need to pretend.

That's not true, Iris, I say, looking straight at her.

We stay still for a few moments, sitting in what we've just defined, in our brackets and abbreviations, in the dead languages we're derived from—the coratĭcums and the cors.

Finally she says, Let's try to come up with a name for the bear. You know how I hate it when things don't have a name.

~⁓

Signora Mirella isn't living in our house; she's renting it out. Or at least that's what my mother suspects after speaking with the doorwoman of the apartment building on Corso Trieste.

That's the house we're supposed to have custody of—legally, it's where we live. But my mother has always feared that the custody would be revoked, that it's hanging by a thread. Her biggest worry, the thing that could break her, is a sudden revocation—someone finding our file and sending caseworkers to check up on us. But the people in charge seem to have forgotten about us all over again. For years now, they've considered us done and settled, like rag dolls in gift wrapping.

Antonia tries to explain it all to me, but it would be easier done with drawings, a diagram—some straight lines, a roof made by joining her hands. Why is it so hard for us to figure out where we belong? To know which address to write on official documents, where our residence is. And if we don't officially reside here, then why are we here in the first place?

Antonia sits by the oven where she's heating up peas and carrots, gesturing in the air and on the table, as if she were packing down bricks or preparing to knead a mixture of flour and eggs. She rolls out and stretches the imaginary dough of our home.

Using her hands and her voice, she starts telling me about how we ended up here, all thanks to a friend of a friend of her friend Vincenzo, the guy who helped us with the move. He mentioned to my mother that there was an opportunity for us—a way to relocate. He had connections. Just a few signatures on some papers, and we could escape. He was the one who orchestrated the house exchange.

Antonia had been miserable on Corso Trieste. We were all unhappy. We faced a new battle every day. We had to defend ourselves from the judgments of all those who had more than we did. She'd spent years fighting for a housing allocation and she was tired, exhausted, ground down. She wanted a calm home, in a calm place.

Vincenzo had spoken with his friend of a friend who knew a woman named Mirella Mancini, née Boretti—a widow who'd been allocated public housing, property of the municipality of Rome but located outside the city, in the town of Anguillara Sabazia.

But Signora Mirella didn't like the lake. She didn't want to live on the shores of anything, and this expulsion from the city weighed heavily on her and her daughters. She was looking for someone willing to swap homes temporarily, without altering any custody or allocation status, but simply by entering into a pact, a private agreement with my mother: Signora Mirella would pay the bills for the apartment in Rome, we would pay for those in Anguillara. She would live on Corso Trieste and we would live in town. And the two of them—Mirella and my mother—would stay in touch to discuss any additional responsibilities. Thanks to a wink here and a nudge there, no one would be checking in on us or giving it any thought.

So my mother, who had always been faithful to her duties and toed the line between legality and illegality, had signed this piece of paper and handed over Corso Trieste to Mirella Mancini, née Boretti.

And now that woman is renting out our house, Antonia tells me, after having summarized the story as best she could. She's renting it out and making money off it because it's worth a lot.

Antonia fiddles with her fingers. She squeezes them until they turn white at the tips, then slams her hand down on the table. She knows she messed up, and she knows that while many people's mistakes are forgiven, ours are not—if you mess up at the bottom, you pay double the price. You have no safety net, no powerful friends, no money to buy your way out.

For weeks, Signora Mirella doesn't answer my mother's calls, or she pretends to be someone else—her sister, her daughter, anyone but herself. When Antonia finally gets through to her, she only tells my mother a few vague things. She says of course she is living on Corso Trieste, or rather, she's letting her daughters live there—no rent, no pranks.

But if your daughters are living there, then you must be living somewhere else—where are you living? The signora says there's been a misunderstanding. She is living there with her daughters—they're all together, of course.

Within a month, the doorwoman assures my mother that she's seen Signora Mirella back in the Corso Trieste courtyard again. Maybe she'd just been away for work or visiting her often-sick sister's house—she has so many sisters, who all live very far away. The doorwoman says she's sorry for having caused us any worry.

My mother lets herself be convinced, and in no time, Corso Trieste fades into the background again—a quietly buzzing concern. I, too, forget all about it.

On December 1, I start decorating the house, launching a full-on campaign to convince my mother that this year we'll be celebrating Christmas properly—there will be desserts, there will be blackjack, there will be a pot roast, and, most importantly, there will be gifts. Mariano and Grandma will join us, and we'll all sit around the same table like saints and coconspirators.

The trees in the park are bare, and with Bear's help, I manage to break off a branch large enough to use as our Christmas tree. He brings a handsaw from home, while I act as lookout. I make sure no one witnesses our crime. The same urge I had as a child to pick the roses sticking out from other people's bushes comes back to me like a slap in the face, but then I turn the other cheek, satisfied with having done something my mother would call indecent.

Bear asks if he can help me carry it home and I say no, I'll do it myself.

I position the branch near the entrance and decorate it with all the red things I can find—socks, ribbons, hair ties, rags, bows, dolls, and I add stars cut out of blank white cards.

Antonia, when she gets home that evening, stares at it and bursts out laughing. She says it's the most hideous thing she's ever seen.

Iris, who's now an accomplice in my mission to reclaim Christmas, finds some old string lights in her grandpa's basement. Not all of them work, and some burn out as soon as we plug them in, but they're enough to create the right atmosphere. We arrange them around the branch and along the edge of our salmon-pink couch—once vermilion, but now faded from my mother's obsessive cleaning.

We're almost there—all that's left are the presents. I immediately think of Luciano's gift to me, which can very well be recycled: it's a bottle-green sweater, twice my size. He had his mother pick it out from their store in the Parioli neighborhood, and she completely ignored the measurements of my shoulders, hips, and waist. It's perfect for Antonia.

For the others, it's a bit trickier. I've never thought about what they like or don't like. I've never thought about needing to please them, about avoiding duplicates in their closets, about putting money aside to surprise them. In the end, Iris's grandma helps us out with some knitted scarves—for Mariano and the twins—and for my father, who would never wear a scarf, she made an orange V-neck vest.

Iris wraps them all in some pages of *il manifesto* that we found in the kitchen drawer, making sure to avoid the ones soiled with lettuce.

As the last day of school approaches, we plan our Christmas break with the idea of meeting up to play cards and tombola, going to the pier, riding the rides, getting offered a glass of prosecco on New Year's Eve—all we want is to recreate the flirty August glances, the shared gossip, the thrill of summer foolishness.

In recent months, we weren't able to see one another very often as a group. The end of the summer snuck up on us, and the start of school swept away the long days at the lake and reading in the sun—everything has changed. I get the feeling we'll never all be together for an entire summer again.

Because of this, Iris and I dedicate ourselves to our holiday preparations with extra care, determined to make everything perfect and bright. We spend hours deciding what we'll wear for the end of the year. Strangely, I'm not bothered by her standing in front of my closet, searching through my limited collection of jackets and sweaters.

This would be perfect for New Year's Eve, she smiles and shows me a T-shirt with the red Superman *S* printed on it, smoothing out its wrinkles from being balled up at the bottom of my closet.

I don't smile. I snatch it from her hands and throw it back where she found it.

That shirt was a gift from Carlotta. She'd bought three of them—one for me, one for herself, and one for Agata. She loved calling us superheroes, talking about our so-called superpowers: flight, mind control, and the ability to turn wood into gold.

I hate that shirt, I snap, slamming the closet door with more force than necessary.

My brother's nose is unfamiliar to me. It's no longer the defining feature of his face, but a common detail, like an ordinary mole or a freckle. His once larger-than-life presence seems smaller to me now, as if I were an adult looking at the furniture and buildings from my childhood—what used to loom large now seems shrunken, as if they were nothing more than harmless moths or beetles.

Mariano is staring at the closet door where I taped some letters cut from Papà's newspapers. I spelled my name out in different shapes and colors, four times over: me, me, me, me. Maybe to make myself like it, to try to think of it as right for me and not just as a label my mother slapped on me, getting it all wrong.

The objects in the room feel distant now, as though Mariano's life has drained out of them. The bed where he used to sleep now holds only the gray shadow of his absence, the faint residue of his being. The sheets of his days are laid out elsewhere. He sits on the edge of his bed then quickly jumps back up, brushing off his pants as if it was dirty or something had contaminated it: our relationship is cumbersome and messy.

Why haven't you gotten rid of it yet? he asks me.

Because it's yours.

I don't live here anymore.

I make a grimace that blunts his frankness, his clear desire to bring me back to reality. To me, the bed is there waiting, always ready for his return, for the night when he'll change his mind and will once again want to divide our room in two with a curtain, to be my other half of this space, look out our window, cast glances and socks into the corners like before.

I heard about your friend, he says, and I notice the small silver hoop hanging from his left earlobe. His face looks like it's aged years, weathered by experience and wind.

Which friend? I ask and grab my brush from the bedside table. I drag it through my hair with determination, preparing myself for Christmas lunch as if it were my first communion.

The one who killed herself.

I don't stop with the brush. Instead, I stubbornly pull it through a clump of matted hair, over and over again, trying to disentangle the knots, to force the bristles and my fingers through.

We weren't friends anymore, I say, trying to liquidate the conversation, make it flow elsewhere, run off into the drainage pipes.

The funeral happened and I didn't go. They planned an event at her high school in her memory and I didn't go. Agata invited me to visit Carlotta's house with her to see her parents and I didn't go. Her death does not exist for me. I avoid her memory because it makes me sick. I resent the unfair feeling of guilt she left me with, I resent the theatricality of what she did, I resent the affectations people have when speaking about it, I resent the hypocrisy of those who suddenly feel a closeness to someone that they never—and I mean ever—loved, and only after her death. I resent how this town seeks explanations for everything, how it investigates young people's deaths in their most intimate and ordinary details: the color of her nail polish, the shirt she was wearing, the size of the bag she used to suffocate herself.

For months, the town has been murmuring and speculating, spinning tales and conjuring demons, retracing every step, forward and backward—how friends like me turned our backs on her, the grades she got in Italian, the dirty and violent messages men sent her, the photos of naked bodies found on her computer, what her face looked like when they found her, how many times she might have masturbated each night before bed. People feast on the dead, sucking out any remaining decency. They pack the funeral just to say they'd been there and they cry for someone they'd felt indifferent toward. Ten, twenty, thirty of them came to me asking why, asking how come, asking how do you feel? And I replied: Great. I'm doing great and I don't know any more than you do.

Now Carlotta hangs over my head like the sword of Damocles or an executioner's axe. She enters my dreams at night to tell me her secrets, then her voice fades away and she turns into a black monster, a harpy, a deep well. Carlotta swallowed up all the secrets—the fake, the real, those never spoken aloud.

But you used to see her a lot, right? Mariano asks. It's probably been really hard for you. Why didn't you say anything about it on the phone? Other people had to tell me.

There wasn't much to say. She died, she committed suicide, and I have nothing to do with it.

I know you have nothing to do with it—what do you mean?

Let's go join the others, I say, abruptly letting go of my brush. Please. Can we stop talking about her now? Antonia's made a pot roast. I've been planning Christmas for weeks.

I hear my voice turn sour and my hands keep smoothing down already smooth strands of hair. I put on the headband I use for special occasions and turn back around to face my brother.

Mariano is an excellent reader. He's always been able to interpret my moods, spot my lost opportunities, but now after all this time apart, I've become a mystery to him. He peers at me, strokes his chin, rises onto his tiptoes. I can tell from his eyes that he wants to slice me open from my throat to my stomach and see what's inside.

I could tell him the truth, one that some people have already figured out: all that's inside me are rocks.

I don't understand you. With those four words, Mariano is asking me what is happening, what's left of me, why I don't rid myself of all these obstacles, why I don't scream or cry, why I have no regrets, whether something is exploding inside me, and, if so, where.

I walk past him and open the door. I hear my mother rummaging around in the kitchen. The table is set, the twinkle lights are on, and my Christmas branch, while far from dignified, is there. It reminds everyone that today is a day of celebration, and each of us must do our best to keep it that way.

My grandma is small in stature and very thin, but she's exacting and efficient. She shadows my mother as she prepares the food and supervises all her movements, from the baking-pan selection to the addition of salt, from the order of the spices to the serving of plates. My grandma says she stopped dyeing her hair years ago because it felt like a waste of money, but she's still a young grandma. If you were to see us from the outside, we all look young—my mother, the twins, my grandma, and Mariano—but underneath, we bear the weight of many long lives. I think she decided to let her hair turn white when Mariano moved in with her; she didn't want to be mistaken for his mother.

Papà! I call him to the table loudly and take a stuffed animal shaped like a rat from Maicol's hands, urging him to sit. Then I invite everyone to sit and light a red candle in the middle of the table with a match. I look around at all of them. We're so unaccustomed to getting together that the table feels tight, the chairs creak.

My father looks like he could start crying at any moment. He has the face of a man who mumbles to himself and tears up easily.

He was surprised to see Mariano, and it made him cling to his fears: he dreads the moment when Mariano will leave again. The silent exchange of glances between nonfather and nonson is tender and almost unnerving. There's affection there, but they don't know how to express it, and they'll never find the words.

Okay, let's start, there's so much to eat, Grandma urges us and serves the food with my mother, handing everyone a plate of baked pasta and advising us to not eat too much of it because we also have pot roast and potatoes and desserts and cheeses. We've gone all out, as is called for.

Our Christmas lasts only half an hour. Just as soon as it arrives, it's over.

What do you mean you don't want to vote? my mother asks.

She's finished her slice of the roast—she'd asked for a small one because she has a boulder in her belly, some nervousness made of stone.

That's it, that I don't want to vote, there's no point, Mariano replies.

The conversations at the table have cruelly shifted away from my brilliant grades, Grandma's canasta club, problems with the electricity at the twins' school, and the fact that Papà wants to throw away all his old neckties, even the green-and-red-striped one from their wedding.

Voting is a privilege, Antonia says and her body is already stiff. I see her jawbone gnawing on nothing.

Maicol says: Can I leave some potatoes on my plate? There's too many.

Everything is a privilege to you, you've been telling that same story forever. Mariano chews with his mouth open, meat juice dribbling out the corners. Voting is useless now, and besides, who should I be voting for?

The ones on the left, Antonia responds and raises her hand, threatening to slap my elbow. Sit up straight, please. You're not the only person at this table.

I take my elbows off the table and stare at the pandoro-cake box. Now seems like a good time to open it, fill the bag with powdered sugar, switch gears, so that's what I decide to do. I stand up and carry my plate to the sink.

Where are you going? We haven't finished the meat yet, my mother shoots a look at Massimo as though asking him to restore order, but he's frozen in place. He was done eating fifteen minutes ago.

Maicol: Can I leave some potatoes?

And who are the ones on the left? Mariano counters.

Well, there are people. Go to your polling place and check, look for Rifondazione Comunista. Will you sit back down? Antonia pingpongs with her words between me and my brother. I start opening the pandoro as a distraction. If I improvised a dance or recited a poem, I'd trick them, get us back to tolerating one another, calm things down.

There's no one left on the left, Ma'. A guy who owns TV channels and newspapers is in power, someone who calls on hookers and looks like a caricature. Mariano snickers, bitterly, and goes back to chewing on that same piece of meat, surely tasteless by now, like cardboard.

I rip open the packaging.

Can't you see we're still on the meat? But if you don't vote, who do you think will govern? How can you complain if you don't even vote? Antonia tries touching my arm to get me to sit back down, and Grandma gestures for me to stop.

Maicol: Can I leave them, Ma'? Can I?

I've joined an anarchist group. Anarchists don't vote. There's other ways to do politics. Mariano swallows his mouthful and washes it down with red wine. He pours more for himself from the bottle in front of Massimo, and to reach the bottle he leans over the table, sticking the edge of his T-shirt into the meat juice on his plate. Then, while drinking, he realizes and dabs at the stain with his napkin.

I rip open the sugar packet. We don't love candied fruit or chocolate at our house, but we sure appreciate powdered sugar.

My mother tosses her fork on her plate but keeps her knife firmly in her hand, using it like a conductor's baton—leading the symphony of her discontent, the rise of her anger.

Ah, great, so after all the protests and the police coming to Grandma's house, now you've decided to set people on fire directly! You haven't forgotten who saved your ass last time, have you? It was me.

Antonia slashes the air with her knife. Her brow is furrowed, pale, and she's sweating from her temples. I know nothing about what's been happening in Ostia. All I know is that Mariano loves the deserted beach clubs that are closed for winter, the sand dunes in Torvaianica, the Kursaal diving board towering above the now-empty pool, and the wooden changing rooms, all torn apart by rain and wind.

That's a bunch of bullshit. You know nothing about anarchy, you know nothing about the left, you know nothing about nothing. You just sit here and give commands like some ignorant saint, thinking

you have a say in everything. Mariano keeps dabbing at the stain with
his napkin, confident that the brown juice will leave his white T-shirt,
as if by magic.

Grandma says what happened with the police wasn't serious,
Maicol asks for updates about his potatoes, and I pour the sugar
into the bag with the pandoro and start shaking it, shaking it
senselessly—I want every inch of the cake to be covered, evenly,
completely.

All I needed was you downplaying it, Antonia says to Grandma,
and then to my brother: I am your mother and I get to have a say in
what you do and don't do. You don't study, you don't work, you don't
vote, and I can't stand your face, it's the face of someone who thinks
he knows everything.

Massimo looks at the half-empty wine bottle, at me, then back at
the wine. If he could run away, I'm sure he would, now more than
ever.

Maicol: Ma', can I leave them?

Grandma, glaring, gestures for me to stop shaking the pandoro
bag, but I don't stop.

I read on my own, I don't need school, and I work at the bar in my
centro sociale. Mariano acts as though he were sitting alone at that
table with my mother. My shaking the pandoro bag doesn't disturb
him, nor does it move him to compassion.

Pum pum, I shake in time with imaginary music, guided by my
sense of rhythm. I'd like to sing something, a church hymn, any
Christmas song.

That's not a job, it's an illegal occupation in some place that's falling to pieces—you think I don't know things? I've been on this Earth

THE BITTER WATER OF THE LAKE · 169

far longer than you and I know places, I know centri sociali, I know who goes to them. Antonia looks down at her fork and potatoes, they've turned dry, tough.

Roberto shrugs at Maicol as if to say he thinks he can leave his potatoes, even though he hasn't received Mamma's explicit permission—it's a bit risky, but he can do it.

Grandma interjects: Mariano does read a lot, that's true.

Do you know what really bothers me? Mariano says. The fact that someone like you, who was involved with neighborhood rallies, housing strikes, protests at the public housing authority, someone who works off the books and cleans the houses of the rich—is telling me what's illegal. Just because something's legal doesn't mean it's right, and you know that.

My mother looks at my grandma as if she was an intruder, the ghost of an enemy slain at war.

Meanwhile I'm running through the list of songs I know in my head, and I realize I don't actually know very many. I don't have a holiday repertoire, nor do I have a good choir voice—my vocal cords are fragile, barely used.

You don't know what it means to be outside the law because I helped you get by. Antonia stands, using her knife to carve angry, invisible symbols in the air. I saved you, I took you far away from that world, and I did it all by cleaning rich people's houses. Anarchy . . . Soon you'll be blowing up packages at the post office. I've never done such things, never, and I fought and I found us a better house, a better place, do you understand?

I keep thumping the cake, now suffocated by the sugar, and I think of Carlotta's face inside a bag—purple lips, wide-open eyes.

Roberto takes Maicol's fork away, silently telling him he can leave the potatoes on his plate, no one is going to be mad at him, and I envy them. They'll always have each other.

We were there with you, don't you remember? Mariano stands up from his chair too, his T-shirt stained, his lips moistened with meat oil, and his nose beak-like as ever. We come from the same place—what did you expect? That we'd wear little bourgeois outfits, go to the good schools, always get up at the right time, become professors? I'm fighting for the same things you fought for. You just don't want to accept that.

Massimo makes a gesture as if to say *let's remain calm*, and my grandma covers her mouth with her hand.

Maicol: Can I leave them? Are we done eating?

I made sacrifices for all of you, you understand? I was just a girl with four kids and no house. I acted like a crazy person for you! My mother's voice is loud but fluid, her words spilling out.

No one asked you to make sacrifices for us, no one! Mariano shouts and his face is deformed by the strain, veins bulging in his neck.

I have to hurry up with this sugar, I have to stop thinking about other things, I have to make it to the end, to save Christmas, to save us all. I shake the bag harder. *Pum pum pum*. The pandoro is starting to break, and the bag feels like it's about to rip open.

Did you want to grow up there? That place was a prison. It was hard to get out, so hard—you can't understand. You don't know what it was like. You should be studying like your sister and looking for a real job—not like mine, not like what your father did—but a real job where they give you a contract, a pension . . . *A real job . . .*

THE BITTER WATER OF THE LAKE · 171

Antonia starts to overflow, but she doesn't sob or wipe her face. Tears start to fall one after the other, forming long lines down her cheeks and above her lip.

Massimo leans the back of his head on the edge of his chair. Grandma still hasn't moved her hand from her mouth.

Maicol: Mamma, what's happening?

This family was done for as soon as we left that place, everything was over, my brother finishes. He pulls us down with him, making us all sink.

The bag finally bursts. Powdered sugar erupts, getting all over the cups and what's left of the meat, the vegetables. It coats the decorations, extinguishes the candles, makes the children sneeze.

The pandoro is on the floor, and no one has opened their presents.

8

What Does the
Lake's Water Taste Like?

I know the town in stages, in encounters, in periods of time: its piazzas, swimming pools, tunnels, its small bridges over narrow rivers, asphalt clearings, the houses in the borgo antico all crowded together, the Piazza del Molo, the lakefront, the Collegiata church, the intersections without traffic lights, the library, the open-air cinema—every place has been discovered, every place belongs to one of the eras of my life.

Now that I have a bike and can ride it on the road, on many afternoons I cross Via Anguillarese and thread my way through the narrow streets of the residential area, pedal past the abandoned house, go down to the soccer fields in front of the hotel with the pool, turn right toward the country roads, and from there head back uphill. I skirt the wall around the hill with its yellow houses and laundromat, emerge at the cemetery, ride past it, and then I decide whether to head into the old part of town or stop at the library. I lock up my bike, walk in, and ask Signora Tiziana if she has anything for me. I don't wait for the library to buy new books in step with the bookstores; I'm used to its damp shelves by now, those in the basement where, awaiting me in the dark, are all of my books.

Even in the coldest months of winter there are bright sunny days when I pull on two pairs of gloves and three pairs of socks and I go out anyway. I ride all the way down Via Anguillarese to the lake, where I pedal slowly past houses with a view of the shore, ivy-covered villas, restaurants packed full on Sundays. I look at the people who've come from Rome to eat fried pike, others stretched out in the meager sunshine, the rowboats tied up on the beach, stones, feathers, drainpipes, the public restrooms (always closed), the railings where children sit, the promenade often teeming with street vendors selling necklaces and terra-cotta vases. Then I turn around and ride back up the hill without even stopping for a coffee. I pass by the gambling house and the gas station, and I keep going, sweaty and out of breath. I could get myself sick.

Thanks to the long hours of boredom and the slow-moving days, I've managed to make this town mine, at least a little bit. I no longer feel as though I've just arrived, too late for the founding myths, the lore, the bedrock.

In this town, people judge you according to your degree of foreignness.

The most beloved and respected people—aside from the doctors— are the ones born into the farming families, those three or four families who have lived here for generations and have land, farms, and stables, who sell meat, olive oil, and vegetables.

Below them are those families that, at some point, chose Anguillara over neighboring towns, roughly two generations back. They don't know the town's oldest stories. They've memorized the names of all the places and know why they're called what they're called, but they weren't the ones to name them. Often they're developers who invested money in the town's boom, transforming it from a village into a small city. Now they own supermarkets and gas stations.

Then there are the people who came from Rome, often middle-class families that grew tired of the city's chaos. They work for companies and public agencies, commute, send their children to schools in Rome, and experience the town like some kind of perpetual vacation. They don't have friends from here and hardly ever stroll along the lake, but they build pools in their backyards and host barbecues under their porticoes or pergolas.

Then there's us: the people who fled Rome because it became too expensive. We live in apartments far from the lake—three bedrooms and a kitchen, small but well-kept living rooms, one car per family (in the best of cases). We often work in town, we find jobs in the shops, bakeries, at the supermarket, or in other people's houses. We open hair salons and stationery stores.

The rich foreigners come next—the Germans, the Dutch, the English—who bought the oldest houses high up in the borgo antico and restored them. They turned them into bed-and-breakfasts or live in them year-round. Some are retired, others started tiny craft workshops, still others work at the Casaccia energy research center as biologists and researchers. They only see the best parts of town: the frescoes in the churches, the sunrise over the lake, the diving off the rocks, the snow-dusted alleyways. They've become some of the least liked, perceived as invaders. The townspeople scoff at their cultural initiatives: the music school, the theater performances, the readings in the piazza.

At the very bottom of the hierarchy—the least loved—are the foreigners who come here looking for simple jobs, or who sell their wares on the sidewalk. They're met with suspicion and sharp-tongued comments. For years, foreign families—Poles, Romanians, and Albanians—have lived in our town, families like mine, people who work hard all day long and who've managed to rent a few rooms. They are construction workers, gardeners, housekeepers, waiters, cooks. All kinds of stories are told about them; the slander spreads quickly.

Agata used to keep me updated on all the supposed crimes being committed by "those people." If a barn roof collapsed, if the streets were dirty, if there was less work being done out in the fields, if a sheepdog got lost, if it was dangerous to go out at night, if beer bottles were found floating in the lake, it was their fault. One of the best rumors was the yearly one about the Romanian man who'd died because he'd drifted away drunk on an inflatable mattress and drowned—the lake had taken revenge.

Agata's paranoia had already been in full force for about a year when she heard that some men, Albanians apparently, were posting up outside middle and high schools to kidnap girls, force them on buses, and drive them to some godforsaken place to be prostituted. Every time we walked out of school, she stuck out her neck and quickly scanned our surroundings. She checked all the parked vans and unknown faces, and she'd ask me: Who is that guy?

When I brought it up to Antonia, asking if it was true, if we were in any danger, she told me it was all nonsense and that we would grow up to be fearful, always waiting for ghosts to appear, unable to react to real dangers, to real crises.

Maybe she was right. Between us girls, we fueled one another's fears, which were magnified by national stories—kidnappings and parents' desperate appeals; girls found dead in industrial zones; the thin, pale thighs of young women on country roads, forced to lure passersby. In our imaginations, trailers on the city's edge became hotbeds of crime and pestilence.

I adapt to other people's fears when necessary. I saw, and still see, my female classmates get consumed by trifles, how they shudder at the first laugh, the first comment said in broken Italian, or at a glance on the street. So, like them, I don't reciprocate; like them, I decide who's an outsider and who isn't, who deserves attention and who doesn't.

After years here, people now know who we are. We exist in this town and are greeted on the street. We've cleaned ourselves up— very little remains to stain us: Mariano's outbursts, Carlotta's suicide, the bear I won at the shooting game. Other than that, they don't really talk about us.

With this new status, this tiny step up, I feel relieved. I'm happy to have established distance from the others and to see that these differences are respected. Let them sink. Let them be blamed for invented sins—what matters is that I'm still here, floating, surfacing.

There's only one bar that stays open at night during the winter, it's in the Piazza del Molo. A couple years ago, it changed management and the new owners renovated everything, replacing the old plastic tables with sleek, modern furniture, adding TV monitors to the tearoom, repainting the window frames, and investing in gelato machines. At first, although the new owners were from our town, their mission to modernize the place was seen with skepticism. But now, after many long, deserted days, their bar is always full, especially on weekends. In the end, they won—partly out of their stubbornness, partly out of our necessity.

It's a Saturday night, and although I'm sitting in the bar, I haven't taken my coat off yet. My hands are frozen from the moped ride and I'm only wearing mascara. I forgot to layer on black eye shadow. I feel naked, exposed to ridicule.

Iris couldn't come out because of an argument she had with her mom, so it's me, Dafne, Ramona, Bear, and the Greco. They're drinking bottled beer and I'm having a soda when some boys Bear knows walk in and start talking about Sunday's Sabazia soccer match. The town has two teams: the first is for people who can really play and who compete in the Eccellenza regional league; the other, the one Bear plays on, is the team of the hopeless, the brawlers, the pigeon-toed, the rejects. On Sunday, they played and lost, and in the locker room after the game the captain punished the goalie by shutting his hand in a locker. One guy held him there while another opened and closed the metal door, over and over again, breaking his fingers.

I was soon bored by the conversation, as I usually am by others' misfortunes. I already have enough of my own thrashing around inside me. I stand up, say I'm going for a walk, and turn down Ramona and Dafne's offers to join.

I shove my hands in my pockets and pull up my hood, the cold humidity rising from the lake passes through me, and I look up to see the lights illuminating the Collegiata above the borgo. I don't often go all the way up there because it's not reachable by bike. The ascents are too steep, the cobblestones are slippery and irregular, and it wouldn't take much to tumble to the ground.

I enter the borgo antico and climb the long stone staircase that, from the Piazza del Lavatoio, leads all the way up to the town hall, where the public library used to be. The building is lifeless and the only sound is the trickling water in the fountain with the two eels. I'm out of breath and there's no one around. The bars are closed and so is the tabaccaio corner store. I follow the lights flooding the church facade.

While I climb, I think about how this is the same path brides take. Every girl getting married in Anguillara wants to do it at the top of the town, in the old church, but for that to happen they have to walk up these narrow streets and alleyways in stilettos. There are so many stories of brides falling, spraining their ankles, and of older relatives collapsing halfway up the hill, under the blazing sun.

I see an albino cat emerge from a side street. Its rosy, bitten ears are practically hairless, its red eyes reflect the streetlamps, and its bright-white coat is like a ghost's. I follow it, straying from the climb. We weave back down among the houses. Many windows are already dark, the clothes that were hanging out to dry have been pulled back inside because the sky was rumbling in the afternoon. The cat runs and stops, runs and stops, and seems to look back at me in the dark.

Patiently, I hurry along so as not to lose it. We pass a staircase overgrown with vines and a painting of the Madonna embedded in a wall. I tread carefully to avoid trampling on pots in doorways or tripping over the chairs old people like to sit in outside their homes. We move deeper into the bowels of the town—its black and antiquated gut—where whispers trail one another behind closed windows and the smell of cellars rises through cracks in the walls.

The cat leaps and bounds soundlessly through this postcard-perfect scene and guides me down the narrowest alleys, the veins running through the borgo antico. My footsteps echo all around me.

Bear told me his grandparents live in the borgo antico and at this point they no longer leave their house; it's too difficult for them to go up and down the stairs. It's hard enough to have them over for holidays or to go see them on Sundays. They've grown used to the isolation and the inconveniences, but from their crumbling, flowerless bedroom balcony, you can see the entire lake and the painted moon.

Where are you running off to? a voice calls out to me and I stop. There's a boy standing outside of a pub. They call it the little grotto because it's a cave that's painted white where they serve dark beers and hot dogs, but we never go there—it always makes me feel like I could suffocate. The walls seem to close in on themselves, and the air becomes unbreathable.

I look around. The cat has disappeared.

I was heading back to the pier, I say, recognizing the boy who spoke to me. I walk toward him.

Why are you wandering around all by yourself? Cristiano asks, first studying me and then the bottom of the bottle he's holding.

What, that's not allowed? I lean against a wall and look at his shadow, projected by the lamplight. Then I look at him: a stick-thin body, long arms, pronounced ears. There's nothing wrong with him, but there's nothing right with him either, nothing tolerable.

There's a madman in the borgo antico who throws things off his balcony, even his iron, whenever he hears any noises under his window at night, Cristiano says, smiling, and sets his empty bottle on the ground.

He starts telling me a story about the time he and his older brothers, along with some friends, stole the key to the town's old gates, the only entrance big enough to let cars into the borgo antico. They bolted it shut for the first time in centuries, then hid to watch the faces of the people who went up to the doors and couldn't figure out how to get through them. He tells me about the times it's snowed, about the flat roofs you can climb onto and navigate from one house to the next, and about the road signs they stole and rode like sleds down the slope to the pier. He tells me how a painter once lived at the end of the lakeshore promenade, where the road is blocked off by a tall fence and a danger sign, and every family in town wanted one of his paintings for their weddings. Each one was worth three months' wages.

And at the top of the borgo, in the house with the largest balcony, lived a female writer who lived with another woman. Everyone knew that they were lesbians, and when they passed by on the streets, the townspeople almost bowed. Then Cristiano tells me about the boy five years older than us who is always roaming around the piazza, in and out of bars, mumbling and lost in his fixations—a fear of lightning, a love for artisanal grappas, for feeding ducks stale bread. He was nicknamed Toro because he was muscular and irrepressible, but then he went on vacation with some friends, took some pills, and came home bloated, slow, off in another world.

And then there's your friend, the bullshitter.

Who?

The Greco. Everybody knows his father's Romanian, not Greek. He's got a hardware store in Manziana.

So?

So he's full of shit.

I shrug. I don't care. I don't even consider him my friend; he's just a boy who's in love with Iris and who I hang out with sometimes. I've never asked him anything about his family or what he thinks of the world. I haven't questioned him about his fears, about what makes him laugh, about why he lies.

What I want to say is that we all lie about our families. They're the lair of our boldest fabrications, where we hide our identities, make up fairy tales, safeguard grievances, stockpile clichés, and barricade ourselves behind the shouting, the screaming, the mysteries—but I don't. Instead, I look at Cristiano and say: Tell me another story.

He nods and we set off toward the pier. I ask if he's ever jumped off it and he says yes, and then: Have you ever thought about the water? They say it's sweet, but that's a lie. It tastes like gasoline. If you put a lighter near it, it ignites.

The winter makes Cristiano seem paler and taller. His hair has grown and it's straight and spiky, kept in place with gel. He's wearing a strong perfume, sugary and raw like citrus juice—it slams against the season's icy air. He still has that sauntering way of walking. He sticks only the tips of his fingers into his jean pockets and his long neck pokes out unprotected from his coat. None of us like wearing scarves, gloves, or hats. Even in February, we show the skin of our hips. We expose our ankles in pouring rain.

Under there, right in that spot, there's a nativity scene with five figurines about this tall. They put it there years ago.

At this point, we're at the end of the pier and I recognize that spot in the water beyond the wooden pilings I'd jumped from, a patch of algae and darkness.

I tell him I know this story and that I've jumped in and swum nearby. I didn't see anything, even though it was broad daylight. He insists that it's really there and that I must not have looked hard enough. The statues are always there, he says, keeping watch over the town every day of the year. By now, they've turned slimy, corroded by the water, yellowed, and neither the currents nor the fish have managed to dislodge them.

When we break away from the railing, I see Bear coming toward us.

I'm leaving, I'll take you home, he says without greeting Cristiano, who I believe he knows.

I can take her, Cristiano offers from behind me, and I nod, telling Bear I'll go with him.

Bear hesitates. He has the same look on his face as he did when he walked down that very same pier to touch the Greco's back and lead him back over the railing. It's the face of someone who protects and knows when to intervene, who can sense trouble, disturbances, and shifts in the current.

After a while, Cristiano brings me home on his moped, speeding as though he's got something against the world. He ignores rights of way, one-way streets, stop signs, intersections. The roads are icy and the tires hiss as he grips the handlebars, contending with equilibrium and his surroundings. He tells me he often turns off his headlights and drives like that in the dark, guided by sound, and he says we'll do it next time—we'll turn off the headlights on the road to Trevignano or the one to Bracciano. He knows all the bends by heart and doesn't need them lit up.

All right, I say.

When we reach my building, I feel the heat rising from the moped. It has blue lights and shiny, beetle-colored paint. Cristiano asks me which house is mine and I point toward our balcony.

Was it you who threw that rock at Andrea's dad's windshield? he asks, looking at me as he plunges his fingers into his pockets and fiddles with his house keys, making them jingle.

No, it was Carlotta Sperati, I say, staring at the knuckles of his other hand, tight on the brakes.

How do you know that?

Everyone knows. People saw her. First she threw the rock, then she went home and killed herself.

When he leaves, I climb the stairs to my house. My mother is awake and has the radio on low. She's knitting. She recently decided to teach herself how to crochet as well. She makes doilies full of holes and floppy hats, devoid of life.

I don't say anything to her. I just wave and signal my presence. I walk over to the house phone, pick up the handset, grab the notebook where I've written down all my useful numbers, dial, let it ring twice, then hang up.

It's a signal to Iris. It means I'm alive and I'm going to bed.

Iris calls Luciano Mama'sprettyboy, all one word, because, as she puts it, he's a big baby who's used to getting what he wants—Sweetcheeks, Babydoll, Angelface. She laughs when I tell her I'm annoyed at how he always repeats the same expressions: *you don't get it, it'll take just a sec, I'm gonna wreck it*—how he calls everyone bro and loses his mind whenever his shirt gets wrinkled.

A story, a relationship, calls for a plot, some characters, something to tell, but I don't have much to say about me and Luciano other than that my annoyance is proportional to his insignificance, proportional to the gifts he's given me, like the one from Christmas—chosen at random, meaningless—and to the hours he wastes talking about AS Roma soccer players, to the scarf he's always folding neatly and carefully placing in his backpack, as if it were a relic, and to his pearly-white front teeth, which look as though they've been sanded down and are full of tiny cuts.

There are periods, entire months even, when we don't talk, when the phone calls to my house diminish and our encounters at school are limited. We choose to avoid each other, yet we never issue the final word, never cut off that connection between two very different people. He clings to me like a mite, he's always there yet I never see him. Then we'll start talking again, about pointless things: our grades at school and our unfulfilled wishes, our ciao ciaos and fake jealousy. He's a master manipulator when it comes to being jealous. He invents reasons to get mad at me and insists and insists on something having happened between me and people I've never even spoken to, on looks I've never received, then he pretends to be stubborn and hurt.

I appear and disappear, often avoiding his demands for attention. I don't engage in conversations about possible betrayals or lies. I'm distinctly uninterested in playing a role in the kind of couple he wants to stage.

I start to believe that this is how relationships work: like shadows.

Making love is a ridiculous expression—it's theater, it's deception. What he and I share, as naked and sentient human beings, is always mediocre. Even from the start, I wasn't able to convert our closeness into any sort of moist sensation. I remained underneath his thrusts, my body silent and my head elsewhere. The lamp on his bedside table projecting light onto our faces. The air coming in from a window left ajar chilling my tingling feet. His breath smelling like half-digested licorice. Outside, the neighbor's dog howling, biting at the hedges. I'm distracted by the life crackling all around us, the life that is not us.

I don't suffer, but neither do I act willingly. I feel aseptic, apathetic, though awake and alert. I don't understand how this ritual could have been passed down through the ages, considered essential.

Usually it's Luciano who initiates and I approach the beginning like it's a bath: I undress, lay out my clothes deliberately, check the water temperature, squeeze in the soap, then climb in, sink to the bottom, and submerge my ears in the water.

I've never asked Iris what she thinks of it. I haven't compared my intimacies with those of my friends, assuming that's how it's meant to be, that all our disappointments should remain private. I've never even asked Luciano what other experiences he's had. I've never asked for ratings or rankings. Stiffly I join him, and stiffly I abandon him.

Mama'sprettyboy makes various attempts to appear appetizing, to animate my desire, to prove himself an expert lover and a cultivator of sensuality. I try to humor him just enough and then return to my own thoughts—the closet doors that could be hiding skeletons, the jeans button rattling in the washing machine, the TV blasting upstairs with lots of shooting sounds—it's a movie where, in the end, only a werewolf is left alive.

One spring afternoon, Luciano walks me to the station after school. He walks farther and farther down the platform, all the way to the end, where the trains don't even reach when they stop. That's where he chooses to pick a fight.

He pulls a piece of paper from his backpack—a letter from a girl older than us, in her final year, who would really like to get to know him. In delicate handwriting, she decorates her interest with paint and rubies. I snatch the note from him and read it, then hand it back without changing my expression. I'm thinking about how the train will be coming soon and how I might miss it.

Luciano isn't happy with my nonresponse, so he passes the letter back to me, telling me to read it again. I open it, glance it over, fold it, and say, I read it. I got it. So?

That sets him off. He launches into a tirade about my lack of love and how I'm withholding the dramatic reactions he thinks I should be having. I should be mad. I should be screaming in response to this threat to our deep bond, to our life together. I should be jumping to my feet and dripping with tears and sweat. The fact that I'm not doing any of this must mean I have feelings for someone else. Who is he, where does he live, is he from your town, does he live near you, is he one of those friends you go out with, the one with the animal name, or no, the one from Turkey, or was it Greece, I can't remember, the one who gives you rides on his moped, one of those peasants who rides a horse around on Sundays, some swineherd?

The train announces its arrival with a mechanical whistle and I can see it coming, its emerald-green snout, the white stripes and the letters *FS*, the round headlights, and the conductor with his beret and dark uniform.

I have to go, I tell Luciano, ignoring his desperate grip on my arm.

He squeezes, not cruelly, but firmly. He insists on me taking the next train—we need to talk, he needs to know. Meanwhile the train brakes and whistles and I try to pull away, but Mama'sprettyboy hangs on tightly as if I were a prosciutto hook and says please, he keeps repeating please.

Agata shouts my name, motioning for me to hurry up and get on the train. I see her blonde ponytail swinging as she calls out to me. But Luciano doesn't let go and keeps saying please, please. I stop pulling away and look at him, my cheeks burning, my bangs disheveled, my legs trembling from the nerves.

What do you have to tell me, can you be quick about it? I yell in his face.

He says he needs five minutes and that we have to work this out. So much time has passed and he can't do it anymore—he can't read or understand me. I was the one who was so insistent on seeing him in the first place, I was the one who said we were soulmates (everyone says things like this, it means nothing), I was the one who demanded his attention, complained about not receiving enough, spent entire afternoons at his house, slept with him, took my clothes off. And yet here I am, giving no weight to our love, no consistency or color.

I hear the signal the train makes when the automatic doors are about to close and clench my fists. The dot on the schedule board next to my train is flashing and so am I. I'm blinking on and off, on and off with rage.

The train departs and passes right by us. It lifts my hair, inflates his shirt, and I think about my friends watching us from the windows, sitting where I usually sit because I'd always rather look outside the train than lay my eyes on the people around me. From the train window, I've seen sheet metal houses hidden among sewer pipes, a private school's soccer fields, construction sites in the hills. I've counted drops of rain. If I stare at my reflected pupils while the train is moving, they dance—right to left, left to right, right to left.

Luciano hasn't fulfilled any of his duties. He's been pale, silent, and fading. He's only rarely brought me any prestige. He didn't elevate my status, didn't bring me into his world or his wealth. I stayed exactly where I was this entire time, not a millimeter forward or back, yet somehow he has the nerve to complain about me, someone who stayed by his side despite the fact that he's so ordinary.

Watching this scene from the outside, I see how much it all oozes with banality—the suicide, the rock through the windshield, the fights at the discoteca, Latin classes, history classes, geography classes, PE. Everything is the same and everything should be thrown away. We're futile animals, worth less than viruses. We're nothing compared to cetaceans, oysters, pachyderms.

What are you even good for? I ask as I see him wavering and losing shape, melting.

He gets mad and says that I'm the one who's good for nothing. I live in my own world fortress, wrapped in my ball of yarn where I hear no words and see no one outside of myself. As for him—people like him, they really do. I think I'm the only one, but I'm not. He sees plenty of girls and they're almost all prettier than me—almost. They're the kind of girls who vacation in Porto Cervo and wear sundresses on moored boats.

I'm perfectly fine with that, I say with contempt.

I feel shame rising up from my thighs about all the times we've been naked together, our fleeting intimacy, my distractions and

ineptitudes, shame about having believed I'd be able to get something out of this when it's clear that the world has nothing for me.

For the first time, the distance between me and Carlotta feels
slight. In the list of Luciano's other girls—their bodies all tanner than
mine, their butts firmer, their bikinis worn with fewer reservations—
I find a place that belongs to both of us: a fragile and cold ravine, the
cave of our desires where we can be admired, not disappoint, stand
out from the rest.

I can't bear this similarity, this proximity to someone who is dead
and shouldn't be showing up anymore—not in my thoughts, not in
my memories, not in my bad habits, not in my dreams. I want to
scream out loud that she's dead and that we had nothing in common.

My hand takes on a life of its own. It sticks out, grabs onto
Luciano's perfectly groomed hair, the object of his endless attention,
and pulls hard.

I don't give a shit about you. Understand? No one betrays me, not
even you, I yell in his left ear.

He bends sideways, caught off guard. For a few seconds, he puts
up with it, unable to comprehend why it's happening, why I would
want to harm him. Then he yells back that I'm crazy, I'm hurting
him, and he pushes me away, saying it was all a lie. He only wanted
to see me react and get upset, but not like this. I'm behaving like an
animal, he says, and should be caged, locked up in chains.

I look at my open hand. His hair falls from my fingers and the
wind carries it away, along with my first love.

Our land is the land of two lakes—ancient volcanic craters that behave like brothers with no ties of affection between them. They have no tributaries in common, no aquifers, no streams. Each lake is responsible for its own water and nothing more.

The second lake is small. You can easily travel from one shore to the other in a paddleboat, and over the years it's become a nature reserve. The only way to reach it is on foot, through the countryside. Cars are left up above, parked between haystacks and stacked wood, and an unpaved descent leads to its shores. Going down, there's a risk of slipping. Going up, a risk of making your heart jump out of your chest.

The smaller lake is called Martignano and it's where young people from town go on Easter Monday, Liberation Day, and May Day. We travel there in groups with our backpacks. Some people bring entire cases of beer, others bring colorful blankets, sandwiches, water, cigarettes, hashish. The bravest stay there overnight. They climb down with tents and camp in the most isolated spots.

The sand is mixed with grass and rocks, it's black and claylike. The water gets deep quickly, and the currents are strong in the middle of the lake. The whirlpools can drag you under.

My favorite spot along the shore is where there's a weeping willow. Beneath it, light filters in with puffs of air, and if I close my eyes, aside from people's voices, I can hear the cows and their bells in the pasture, the chimes they make when they move.

That's where Cristiano says he first saw me, on May 1 of the previous year, the same day I met Iris and the rest of the group.

We were lying in the sun, we future friends, and were all wearing cheap plastic sunglasses. It was the first time our winter-pale bodies were being exposed to the world, with purple circles under our eyes and blue veins decorating the tops of our feet.

Our small talk was awkward and truncated. We didn't know one another yet, so we asked questions and shared insignificant details about our lives: school, our town, the recent Easter holidays, summer plans.

Not far away, another group had formed—a few girls and many boys, some our age, others older, all from our town. After a couple of hours, they had finished their cases of beer and were drunk. They played soccer on the beach, hitting bystanders with the ball, they laughed and cursed, throwing themselves on the ground and rolling toward the water, making faces, and speaking in dialect—both among themselves and about us.

The mood of the group quickly shifted, from carefree to aggressive. They shouted insults and threw empty cans at one another. Some vomited on tree trunks, and the families with children sitting nearby got up one after the other to move farther away or head home. Two of the boys, best friends and schoolmates, started fighting—though no one ever figured out why. Their boisterous laughter turned into blame, and blame turned into murderous glares. Then they starting going at each other like feral dogs.

Their friends, drunk and dizzy, tried to stop them, grabbing them by their shoulders and begging them to calm down. Some saw the confrontation as a game and formed a circle around the contenders, urging them toward destruction. A crowd gathered and I, too, went over to watch. They were hitting each other savagely. On their skin you could already see signs of the punches they'd exchanged.

When the blood came, I pushed my way through the onlookers to get a closer look. Their faces were covered in red: one had a broken nose and the lip of the other had split open.

Cries of concern grew louder. Their girlfriends stood at a distance, sobbing, leaning on their friends, terrified of the evil that had erupted and that no one knew how to contain. The adults had dispersed. We were left all alone with this tragic scene.

The more they tore each other apart, the closer I got. I stayed until they'd both crumpled to the ground, exhausted from the brawl and the alcohol. Their faces were unrecognizable, their eyes shut, their hair sweaty and matted with blood.

Their friends came to their aid once the fight was over, pulling them up by their arms and legs, and only then did I realize I was the only girl still standing there. My friends had all moved away. They'd gathered up the blankets and backpacks and had gone to seek refuge beyond the willow, putting distance between themselves and the fight.

I turned around, searching for them, and felt unfamiliar and curious eyes on me. Who knows if anyone recognized me as the girl who knew how to shoot, the daughter of Antonia the Redhead, the girl who loves carnage, bloodshed, and nasty wounds.

That's when Bear came up behind me, grabbed me by the wrist, and led me away: They're idiots, a bunch of idiots, he said, keeping his open hand on my bare back.

I was there that day, too, Cristiano confesses, one of those boys was my brother. He had a broken capillary and banged up his head, but nothing serious. He's doing great, he tells me, and with his short fingernails he scratches some grime off his moped's handlebars.

I've always wondered why you stayed, he asks, looking up at me.

To watch, like everybody else, I say and rest a foot on his front tire. I push it as if to make him lose his balance. He straightens himself out and puts down his kickstand.

Not everybody, Cristiano clarifies and we're silent for a moment. Kids can be heard playing soccer in the background. We're near the station and behind the church.

What did we come here for? I ask and move my foot.

I have to ask you something.

So ask it.

I recently found out that this is the church for funerals, which means we get married at the top of our town and we say farewell in the lowest part, farthest from the lake. We're joyful among the stuccos and the frescoes, the old wooden altars and the sacred smell of stones, well-dressed and perfumed, and we cry in front of the modern, diamond-shaped stained glass and the toxic air of an obsolete faith. Where the pews form a semicircle and the priest looks like he's presiding over a conference, with the same enthusiasm he might show in a lecture hall. We always die in the shittiest place, where we're miserable, shabby, and washed-out. We disappear while the priest forgets our names, and not even Christ's face looks the same anymore.

I need some information, Cristiano says, growing serious. He climbs off his moped and comes closer, speaking more quietly.

He asks me if it's true that I go to a rich-kid school, and I nod, then he asks if I have friends who live in the neighborhoods at the end of Via Cassia, and I say I don't have any friends there. He asks if I know anyone, though, if I've seen their houses, and I say maybe, then he asks which house and I tell him which house. He asks, What do they have inside? Plasma televisions? Jewelry? Designer handbags? I say yes, two TVs—one on the ground floor, one in the basement with the new PlayStation. The closets with the purses are on the second floor, in the bedroom on the right. There's a safe but I don't know

THE BITTER WATER OF THE LAKE · 195

how to open it. He asks if there are any alarms or guard dogs. I say I don't think so—they only have a small dog, but the neighbor's dog is always barking.

He pulls a piece of paper and pen out of his pocket and asks me to write the address on it and whatever I know about the people's schedules. I take the piece of paper and turn it over in my fingers, thinking about their schedules. I write down the time they leave the house in the morning, more or less, where the mother works, where the father works, the time they come home. I know they have a cleaning lady—she's Filipina. She comes in at ten and leaves after lunch, so there are three empty hours. I underline them: from seven to ten in the morning. But before handing the paper back to him, I ask what I'll get out of it and what the risks are for me.

Cristiano says I'm not risking anything and I can have whatever I want—so, what do I want?

It's the first time anyone has ever asked me this question. Until now, no one has ever offered to fulfill any of my desires. Everyone has always assumed that I'm happy as is, that I have nothing to ask for, that there's nothing missing from my life. I think about it for a full minute and then say that there's one thing I want: a cell phone, any cell phone, but I need someone to set up the phone plan for me—I can't ask my mother for one.

Cristiano says it's no problem, am I sure that's all I want?

I could tell him that I want everything—everything in that house and in the house next door, all the cars parked on the street, all the mopeds in every garage, all the television antennae, the stand mixers, the electric ovens, the purses, the immersion blenders, the couch pillows, the bathroom rugs, the cupboard doors, the geranium pots in the back, the roof tiles—but I say yes, that's all I want, and I surrender the piece of paper, adding that I don't know any other houses, so they shouldn't come asking me for more.

He says that's fine. This isn't something they do often, but right now they need money. I don't ask who they are or why they're short of funds. I assume it's none of my business.

In the basement closet there are at least twenty blue Ralph Lauren sweaters, in case you like them or want to sell them, I add and put on my helmet. Now take me home. I have a Latin test tomorrow.

He nods and gets back on the saddle, kicks up the stand, and has me climb on behind him.

Two weeks later, the news spreads at school: People broke into Luciano's house and took everything. They repeat *everything* as if it were a sacrilege: everything, everything, everything. No one saw a thing. Who knows how they knew his house would be empty? Maybe they'd been waiting outside the gate, maybe they'd followed the family around for months, hidden inside a van. The cleaning lady was fired on the spot—because, you know, you can't trust these Filipinos. They seem well-bred, they seem like good people, they seem to want to work, but turns out they're just like all the rest.

Agata says she hasn't been sleeping well ever since she heard the news. She's afraid someone will break into her house, too. She noticed a car parked on their street a couple of times. It was red and it had a license plate that was not Italian but from someplace like Bulgaria, Moldova, Russia.

I tell her: You're right, it was probably one of them. Better be careful.

9

Forbidden to Minors

For years, all I did was save phone numbers in my contacts, come up with nicknames, press the keys to select the different letters, write text messages in the middle of the night, wake up from nightmares—one of many mechanical sharks decided to eat me, of all people—open it up like a shell, and make it shine. My Motorola, which has already gone out of fashion because it's not in color, doesn't have the internet, and doesn't take high-definition photos. My Motorola, which I tried to hide from my mother, between my thighs, but she still found it. She insulted me and wanted to know where it came from and why, what I needed it for at my age. I had to say it was a loan and then a gift, then I had to hide it better, shut it inside a shoebox.

For years, all I did was take the train—direction Viterbo, direction Roma Ostiense—run so I wouldn't miss it, open and close the ashtray, scratch the seat fabric, block the doors with my body to keep them from closing, shove whoever got too close to me, stare coolly at a woman who'd fainted in the bathroom from the heat, insult whoever it was who'd gotten sick two compartments from mine—it's their fault we're stopped between Olgiata and La Storta, waiting for first responders—and despise that employee whose business was shuttered, leading him to kill himself at the Balduina stop.

For years, all I did was study and review, underline, take notes, draw, transcribe, articulate, get interrogated, receive grades, receive reprimands, receive praise, lug dictionaries, translate from Greek, from Latin, from English, from Old Italian, paraphrase, do logical analysis, do grammatical analysis, memorize poems, declensions, and pronouns, fill notebooks with conceptual maps and notes, arrows and question marks, outline tasks for the following day, yell that I need silence at home to study—silence.

For years, all I did was go to the library; bring books in and carry books out; hide the late returns, the stains, the careless dog-ears; hate, coexist with, rediscover characters, settings, furniture; force myself to learn; skip the pages I didn't understand; drag out impossible and hostile readings; keep lists of what I read so I wouldn't forget; and dream about the day I'll have read everything—absolutely everything—so no one can tell me I don't deserve a reward for this, some kind of honor and attention.

For years, all I did was lie, argue, fight, express myself wordlessly, throw tantrums, make amends for show, make demands, feel mocked, challenge every critic, every disgrace, every neglect, make and lose connections, recover them, lose them again, forget my mistakes, love my mistakes, tell myself I'm grieving, that I suffer constant affronts, that everyone should respect me, include me, tolerate me.

For years, all I did was cover myself up, avoid nudity, avoid ostentation, and stay far away from other people's bodies, not because I'm good—there's no goodness in me, nothing chaste or pious, nothing uncontaminated—but because naked people fill me with dread, the having to please them, not knowing how to approach them, their smells, my smells, the mouths they open, the lips they moisten, the breathy words they say.

For years, all I did was go out at night, always to the same places, where the same bodies sway and the same faces smile or glare at one another; climb into the car of someone I'd just met; end up at a discoteca in the countryside near Viterbo; resent the violet lights projecting bruises on my skin; end up on a partially paved road in a speeding Audi that swerves off it, skidding into a barn and knocking it down; throw myself into the lake's water—headfirst, backward, pencil diving, cannonballing, off of somebody's shoulders, from the wooden pilings by the pier, from a paddleboat platform; scrape my fingers with broken glass from a bottle left on the beach; get my calves covered in blisters from the chemicals somebody dumped into some sewage or canal.

For years, all I did was pedal downhill, uphill, along sharp bends, to the supermarket, to the post office, to where my mother works, to the twins' school, to the tabaccaio, to the pastry shop, to the fruit-and-vegetable market, to the train station, to the library, to the intersection, to the lake.

For years, all I did was stand guard while someone stole money from the slot machines in a bar; ruin the paint of some cars with a key; use spray paint to write the name of a professor with *jerk* next to it because he gave me a B instead of an A on the science test; use a moped helmet to hit some asshole in the face who tried forcing me to drink a beer with him, making blood gush from his nose.

For years, all I did was get dressed, get undressed, recoil at my own skin, cherish my hair, hide my hips, find fault with my ears and my long feet, pull on my nipples to make my breasts grow, punish myself if I ate too much, shame myself if I didn't eat at all, skip breakfast, clean my ears with jets of hot water, paint polish on my fingernails, finish the mascara, drop the foundation in the toilet and wipe it off with toilet paper, check that my freckles aren't visible, get sunburned in the summer, let a rash spread on my chest, go swimming with a T-shirt on.

For years, all I did was hear reports on the radio about robberies, murders, serial killings, bombings, avalanches, earthquakes, super-lotto winnings, soccer-championship winnings, Mafia trials, fallen governments, stabbed children, excessive heat, excessive cold, raped students, departing soldiers, police convoys, hacked banking data, media blackouts, the Sanremo Music Festival.

For years, all I did was listen to people talk about the school janitor who stares at female students; about the ugly, mustached twins who always walk in a pair and share the same Albanian boyfriend; about the gas station attendant who waters down the gas and sells it for less; about the girl who studied international law abroad but is now the mistress of a married man; about the boy who gets girls pregnant, then leaves them and who doesn't even know the names of his children; about the waitress at the bar who's become so anorexic you can see her cheekbones; about the two teenagers who were killed when riding a moped without helmets on a rainy day; about how much weight the girl who was once the prettiest in town has gained (you marry them and then they turn into cows, putting on ten kilos just in their butt); about my dead friend who suffocated herself, suffocated herself, suffocated herself, your friend, your dead friend who suffocated herself. I hope I'm not next in line.

For years, all I did was wait for revolutions, landslides, chain reactions that would lead to my ascent, to an unfolding of infinite possibilities.

For years, all I did was stay where I was—same place, same time, same role, same face—waiting to turn eighteen like one would wait for a prophecy, the arrival of a storm, the fall of a wall.

There's a man and he needs to burn. He's made of straw and is wearing a jean shirt and a pair of corduroy pants.

They pulled him out of a van, one person holding him by the head and the other by the feet, the hay stuffed inside two rubber boots. It's good luck, they say. He represents the passing year, which will go up in flames.

I'm wearing a sequin-covered dress—it's Agata's. It's too short on me, and while I walk around in the piazzale it rides up, almost revealing my underwear. I keep pulling it down by the seams, but it keeps riding up again. I pull it down, and it rides up. I pull it down, it rides up. My jacket is open and the cold goes straight to my head. Meanwhile, the boys have come back with the gasoline.

This night is all my fault—I willed it into being. When Agata asked me two weeks earlier what I was doing for New Year's Eve, I said: Nothing, I think, it's just me and Iris. So she invited us to spend it in a vacant storefront her boyfriend's dad owns. It's where they'll soon be moving the family business, but for now it's empty and we can use it to celebrate.

Iris was doubtful at first. We don't know anyone, she said. We could call Bear and see what those guys are doing, she added, and I reminded her that we haven't seen Bear in months. That friendship—seasonal, sincere, real—ended as only the truest things can end. Now we're distant, for one reason or another. There were no specific blowups or schisms; we just drifted apart. What's left is me and Iris, and our space is the only space I know how to inhabit. Our perimeter is a bunker and a bomb shelter. Outside there are wars and conquests, gamma rays, floods.

I convinced her to go to the party because the thought of trying to get some other invitation by calling around and begging for attention made me want to throw up.

Cristiano left town for the holiday. He rented a farmhouse in Tuscany with his brothers and friends. They went as a pack, bringing alcohol, large quantities of pasta and ready-made sauce, a package of lentils to eat after midnight, and three traditional cotechino sausages.

We weren't invited.

Three hours before the party, we met up with Agata at her house, in her attic bedroom with its mustard-yellow walls and full-size bed. She has a built-in wardrobe and a full-length mirror next to her dresser. Agata and Iris have met on occasion, but the tracks of these two friendships have never truly crossed; they've always run parallel in my life, until tonight.

I watched them choose the outfits they'd wear—blouses, tops, shorts, skirts—and lend each other different cosmetics, pulling them out of colorful cases, styling each other's hair with a curling iron, enthusiastically showing off the lucky red thongs they'd be wearing, putting glitter on their eyelids, exaggerating with lip gloss, raising the volume on Agata's stereo, dancing around, and chatting as though they'd always had many things in common.

Iris loves horses and goes three times a week to stables outside of town, but she can't afford her own horse or lessons with an instructor. So in exchange for riding and training, she helps tame the frisky horses. She curries and brushes them, makes sure they always have food and that their stalls are clean. She also teaches classes for children, and organizes outings for rich American ladies, taking them on horseback through the woods near Lake Martignano.

Agata comes from a farming family. No matter how hard she tries to forget it and detach herself from their rural ways, they remain stuck to her. Everyone knows her father and has a clear idea of what her future will be: taking over the bookkeeping for the family business, a return to her roots. She'll have to stop posturing as a rich bourgeois. But tonight, Agata gets to boast about her family inheritance: the horses they ride through the fields on the weekends, the types of saddles they use. They aren't into dressage or obstacle jumping, like Iris is. They prefer Western riding and ranch life; they own pigs, geese, and mares.

I soon walked away from the conversation, distancing myself from their sparkling outfits and the polish on their nails. I felt microscopic, worthless, a mere conduit for what seemed to be an inevitable friendship. I nursed this strange sensation for the entire night: an intercostal strain, a hole in the spleen, the insatiable desire to begin all over again, starting with that request about New Year's Eve. I wished I could change my answer and tell Iris we'd be alone, just the two of us, at my house, with my father who celebrates by getting drunk (his one night a year) and my mother who wears her red sweater and dances in the kitchen with the twins, both looking entertained and carefree and alive. I can't stand them.

They were talking about the bridles, the riding cap, the different kinds of boots, how many horses there are in the stables, how high do you jump, how often do you ride, have you ever tried to ride bareback? We could go together, next Saturday maybe.

Meanwhile, I kept applying eyeliner, smudging it with every touch. Glimpsing my reflection in the mirror, I looked like a supporting character clamoring to get noticed. There wasn't a thing about my face that was recognizable. My mouth was swollen from the lipstick, and my hair knotty and puffy, like infected gums. It looked like a meteorite had exploded in my face.

We're going to be late, we've been here for two hours and you guys still aren't ready, I said irritably, a jealous edge to my voice, as I gathered up my discarded clothes and stuffed them into Mariano's black backpack.

I know nothing about animals—not cats, not dogs, not ducks, not herons, not flamingos, not giraffes, not horses. Even when they're in books, they bother me.

What a terrible photo, I said, pointing at a frame on a shelf.

It's one taken with a disposable camera, of me, Agata, and Carlotta sitting on a bench at the station. That's how we looked: used and disposed, crumpled, depleted, ready to be recycled.

There are at least two dead people in the photo, and one of them is me, I thought. My twelve-year-old body double who hates her ears, loathes swimming in the pool, and is being harassed by a boy with curly hair. The girl whose racket strings are still intact, who isn't yet full of malice. She makes me feel both pity and repulsion. She and I are as distant as the stars—a journey from here to Saturn.

I like it, I think we look nice, Agata said and then changed the subject, waving four or five perfume bottles in our faces, offering to pick one out for each of us. The bottles went *clink clink*, and I stared at them like they contained pesticide.

Now I'm here with some perfume on my skin that smells of cream and candies, while the straw man burns—and with him, the year 2005. Surely 2006 will be a lucky year, the astrologists all say so, they read it in the stars: a year of love and health, of amazing, unforgettable beauty.

We ate pizza and french fries for dinner at a makeshift table and drank Peroni beer and bottles of wine stolen from our families' cellars. I supplied a box of cheap Tavernello, to everyone's horror.

Agata's boyfriend is the son of the florist. He has a square jaw, a large face, and perpetually tanned skin. He's learning how to make floral arrangements, cut stems with precision, decide which tulle to choose for each bouquet, and how to convince customers to buy the more expensive roses.

That's how I found myself eating with at least ten people I know only by name and who I'd never wanted anything to do with. Three of them spent the night staring at me.

You're Scherani's girlfriend, right?

And I said no, Cristiano and I aren't dating, we aren't friends, we aren't anything. Now he's in Tuscany, he abandoned me here at this beautiful little party where the topics of conversation are spring flowers, galloping horses, and how much cocaine to snort in the bathroom after midnight.

The straw man was propped up against a woodpile. He could barely stand and kept falling over on his side. It took them half an hour to find the right position for him. Then they soaked him with a gray can of gasoline, told everyone to stand back, and started the countdown.

Iris came up to me smiling, her hands under her armpits because of the cold. She wants to say *Happy New Year* to me first, she tells me, and I tell her I can't wait for it to all be over—the year and us and this pageant of clowns and nobodies.

Now she's distant and hostile. I'm provoked by her gaze, her sickening flattery. I'm quick to recoil and grow cold, at the very moment when our friendship is in danger and someone more alluring than me is set to ensnare her. I don't know how to make myself pleasant. I can't disguise myself as a patron saint. Instead, I spit flames and build walls around me.

We can hear the fireworks going off in the countryside and over the lake. The straw man catches fire and we watch him burn and die out— the shirt, the pants, the rubber boots. Some dance around him—the pagan ritual for rebirth—strung out on marijuana and pills. They hop around and wave their arms to the black sky. They pop the corks off bottles of prosecco, shooting them into the air, and the girls all scatter, squeaking like hamsters, so the spray of alcohol won't get them wet.

The left side of my head gets soaked because I'm still standing there, staring into that fire, totally absorbed. We're the only people in the piazzale. One of the boys is lying on the ground, getting his picture taken with a compact camera while draining an entire bottle on his own, and Iris is no longer by my side—she's gone off to toast with Agata and the other girls. They look one another in the eyes while blowing kisses and clinking glasses.

I take my cell phone out of my jacket pocket. Cristiano texted to wish me a happy New Year. I don't reply. Instead I think to myself: he should die, he should die, he should disappear.

Then my phone vibrates again and another message pops up: *Happy New Year, I've been thinking about you.*

I don't recognize the number and assume it's a joke. I write back: *Who is this?*

My cell phone is silent for a few minutes, then another message appears: *Andrea.*

I see the name and immediately think about how much I want to get away from here—away from the straw man, from Iris and Agata laughing, from the boys who have already gone back inside and are arranging lines of cocaine on the table where we'd eaten. One line a head brings abundance, success, and riches.

I type: *I'm in the parking lot in front of the post office, this party sucks, come get me?*

He responds almost instantly: *Yes, I'll be there in ten.*

I look over at Iris with her black hair and pointy boots, the plastic cup in her hand, and she feels so far away, like a silhouette disappearing into fog.

My mother wants to extend her dominion from my childhood into my adulthood. For weeks, I've been telling her no—I don't want this milestone to be celebrated in any way. I don't want to get dressed up for the resurrection, I don't want my picture taken when my transformation is complete.

Since we never celebrated Mariano's eighteenth birthday, Antonia thinks she'll save her soul and get herself reinstated in the pantheon of good mothers by organizing a party for mine, against my will, to my detriment.

Massimo is increasingly nervous about her plan because it also involves him. He'll have to come dressed up nicely and neatly combed, stop coughing and spitting, leave the tube of zinc oxide we use for his wounds on the nightstand, wear shoes instead of slippers, and be presented as the head of the family. He'll be forcibly hoisted into the elevator and dragged outside where the light of the world can illuminate him.

My father moves around the house with an unusual slowness in the days leading up to the party, and it seems as though he's making his wheelchair squeak on purpose, opening doors as if weighed down by some ancestral fatigue, forgetting how to reach the sink or his ashtray, dragging himself around like a phantom.

I said it countless times and in every way possible—there's nothing worse than a party organized by your mother that your father feels forced to attend. Still, Antonia quashed all my complaints with her pointed looks and her inexplicable enthusiasm.

She pulled her nice dress out of her closet only to find—with theatrical frustration—that it was too tight on her hips. Thus began the race for our party dresses.

I made it clear that I'd be useless, incapable of evaluating fabrics, eyelets, colors, sizes, or slits up the thigh. Taking refuge in my room, in the protective shadow of my pink bear—guardian of my adolescence—I rejected any attempt to get me involved.

It didn't work: a short red dress appeared on my bed, made of some flammable, lightweight material, department store style, without shoulder pads, and with seams in another, lighter shade of red, visible and clumsy. That was Antonia's gift to me: a dress for my last day as a child, something glitzy to wear as my introduction to everything forbidden to minors.

Isn't it beautiful? she asks me, leaning against the doorframe, and I say no. A girl with red hair can't wear a red dress. It'll make me look like a torch, like a firefighter.

She doesn't abandon her primal, incurable joy. Instead she circles around me, takes the dress, and holds it up to me. She exclaims glee-fully and calls the twins in to see.

Maicol and Roberto, in all their goodness and simplicity, say it will look great on me and, as they often do, they back each other up. One says *really good* and the other says *really, really good*. One looks at me and smiles, the other nods and claps his hands: Red is definitely my color.

I can't stand their common purpose, the way they manage to embrace my mother's every plan. They're beginning to get zits on their faces and to assume the same polite placidity of a spring day.

Papà really doesn't need to come, I say, looking at the wall because I don't have a mirror in my room and their eyes are the only judges.

Of course he's coming, Antonia replies and urges me to try on the shoes. They're in a box, they have low heels—the kind of shoes only mothers would buy for their daughters, rounded and made for dancing the Charleston. I stare at them, depressed, and push the box away with my foot.

I want to be happy, I just want to be happy, let me be freaking happy! I feel like screaming, but I can't. I send them out of my room and try on the red dress and the shoes. They're too tight on the toes of my right foot. There's nothing to hide behind, nothing to mask my misfortune.

My mother comes back in and says she's really pleased. I look like a movie actress, she says, and I remind her she never goes to the movies. How would she know what people in the movies look like?

The party is held in one of the rooms of the gym near our house. My mother has covered some shifts for the woman who cleans there and became friends with the owner. He's letting her use the space for free so long as she cleans it the following day. It smells like sweat and terry socks. Colorful lights hang awkwardly in the corners. There's a table against the wall with green plastic cups, plates, forks, and sandwiches, several bottles of wine, a lot of Fanta, and pineapple juice. A bald man, the father of one of my neighbors, is the DJ for the night. He decided to kick things off with Latin American dance music.

If I wasn't the birthday girl, I'd be looking for a way out.

It took three people to carry my father's chair into the gym because there aren't any access ramps, and he had two panic attacks: the first in the elevator of our building, the second when he discovered that an entire universe exists, that there's life outside our front door, people walking, people breathing.

I still don't understand how my mother came up with the guest list. Most of the people I know are here, almost all the boys and girls my age. They say ciao ciao and happy birthday, kiss my cheeks and compliment my dress and makeup, breathe into my ear that I've grown up and they're glad to see it.

There are four women standing near the buffet table: the hairdresser who's had a perm since '86 is pouring the drinks, the cashier from Antonia's favorite grocery store is handing out plates, the fishmonger's mother is serving the guests shrimp with pink sauce, the owner of the train-station bar—her hair stiff with three tons of hair spray—is folding napkins into little origami swans, beaming as she hands them out.

Antonia shines, embracing everyone. Seeing her in makeup and a black dress, I find her beautiful. Her breasts are noticeable and her ankles look elegant. While my mother is reborn, I wither away.

Massimo found a secluded corner where he can be embarrassed in peace and have brief, strained conversations with all the people who feel obliged to come say hello, who lean over or kneel in front of him. He hopes no one notices the portable urinal he'll have to use and keep with him until the party ends.

It's nine o'clock and the summer night has just fallen.

Iris is in that yellow dress she was wearing the first time we met. Her hair is tied up in a high ponytail, like Agata's. They're walking toward me together and I can no longer distinguish between past and present. I feel the sting of a slap. There's one blonde and one brunette, balanced and desirable. They're wearing the right colors, they know how to walk on heels taller than mine, and they've applied the same peach-colored lipstick.

I soon discover that they were the ones who helped my mother. They invited everyone we know and did their best to get everyone to come. They approved the menu, said yes to the music, and vetted my dress and shoes, deeming them suitable. Together, they prepared the pastry cream cake exactly how I like it. Hours and hours of subterfuge behind my back. They even made a poster for me, and once everyone arrives, they pull it out. It's orange, and it has photos pasted to it: many of me and Iris or me and Agata in different phases of my life, and others where I'm alone. There's one of me as a baby, wide-eyed, wearing my brother's T-shirt, my face covered in tomato sauce, my feet planted on the concrete of our first home's courtyard.

My tormentors take pride in pointing out the photos they chose and the words they wrote out for me: poems about friendship, famous quotes, all found online and stitched together into a collage of our fictions. Iris's eyes glisten as she reads off all the reasons she loves me. She made a list in the bottom right-hand corner of the poster. It says I'm intelligent, dependable, loyal, and courageous.

The very last word hits me like a punch to the face. It invalidates our bond and nullifies all my past confessions. I don't want to be any of these things. I don't want adjectives to describe me, I don't want people's tears, I don't want parties or posters. My brackets are empty, I don't have Latin roots, Sanskrit roots, French roots. I don't have prefixes or suffixes. I'm a missing definition.

I look at them and don't know what to say. People clap, and everyone talks about how it's such a tender and kind gesture. I say thank you and hug them stiffly. My stomach feels like steel, my joints are rigid, and I smile with the same effort it'd take me to walk across the entire city.

I want to burn that poster and watch it go up in smoke. I wish I could go home and cut it into tiny, ingestible pieces.

Other people come up to me, handing me gifts and cards, and I look around, searching for my brother. I'm convinced he'll show up, shut off the music, give everyone a slap on the wrist, and make them realize they're hurting me. But Mariano doesn't show. People keep coming and going, and the gifts pile up in my arms.

Ma', where's Mariano? I ask my mother, my eyes desperate. She tells me she didn't invite him.

The music is loud, and my friends tell me to put the gifts aside and come dance. Ramona, Marta, and Dafne are there too, along with everyone who rides horses with Iris, the whole majorette team, the children of the people my mother works for, some of the boys from my class in their short-sleeved linen shirts. Carlotta's sister approaches, kisses my cheek, and says, This is from Carly. She would've wanted to be here, I'm sure of it. Then she starts tearing up.

No, she wouldn't have wanted to be here, and in fact, she's not. Look around—does it look like she's here? Does it? I want to yell in response, but I'm overwhelmed by the realization that no one has bothered to understand what would be right or wrong for me. No one has thought about what I really want. Everyone's just playing their roles, following the script of all eighteenth birthday parties—full of good intentions, farewells to youth, and renewed promises.

None of this feels legal or legitimate to me.

My friends let out a cry of excitement, they're pointing at some-one behind me. I can barely breathe. I want to throw myself to the ground and squeeze my eyes shut. But I turn around, urged on by their gleeful faces, by their wide, eager smiles.

Andrea has entered the room. He's wearing elegant trousers and a dress shirt, and he's carrying a bouquet of roses. His face is clean-shaven, his hair styled, and his handsomeness is just another source of discomfort on top of everything else—the way he walks, his sol-emn movements, the fresh roses in his hands. Without any hesita-tion, he comes straight up to me and kisses me. I feel the moist lips of our past against my broken mouth. People are applauding. My mother exhales with satisfaction—such a good boy, such a dear and honest boy.

And that's when I understand why Cristiano isn't here, either. No one invited him. Or, more likely, they told him not to come. My mother and my friends don't think he's suitable for my new life, for this saintlier, more perfect version of me.

The message is suddenly clear: there has to be a new me. The old me—reckless, violent, prone to making scenes—is now part of the past, archived with my youth. Starting today, I have to clean myself up, wear my best smile.

I take the roses and hold them against my chest. I look into Andrea's eyes and realize that not a single person here knows me as I really am. No one here knows about that night I hurled the rock at his father's car before heading to the discoteca, to communicate that nothing had been forgotten, and that he would continue to pay.

I should tell him it was people like him who killed Carlotta. He and all the others—the ones who cleared their consciences by showing up to the funeral, but who would have been ashamed to be seen getting a gelato with her when she was alive. The boys from the back rooms and the dark corners and the behind-the-scenes, the ones who said, Touch me, but stay behind me, I don't want to see your face.

Andrea squeezes my side and whispers for me to set down the flowers. The time has come, he says, to dance like only adults know how.

My Italian teacher looks up at me from below, wearing a leopard-print overcoat that nearly touches the ground. Her bowl cut doesn't even move when she sneezes. She asks what I plan to do with my life—start working, right? She repeats my last name twice as if I weren't standing right in front of her and asks me again. You could do a certification course. What about graphic design and communication? What about joining the army? What about nursing? It only takes three years to become a nurse and in hospitals they pay right away. Or maybe you could be an aesthetician, or a secretary in a law firm? I don't see you as an athlete, swimming, running—do you have any skills? She pulls an anise-flavored candy from her pocket, sucks it, then dislodges it with a fingernail when it sticks to her teeth.

I reply saying I don't know yet, I still need to think about it. Her face clenches like she's trying to wring water from her cheeks.

There's one month to go before the nationwide high school finals—the dreaded maturità exams—and I'm studying even while the others sleep. By day, I'm an evanescent presence—eyes red, open wide, and glued to the blackboard. I underline pages in my books almost until they tear. Even Antonia says I'm overdoing it. She knocks on the bathroom door and threatens to call the fire department when I fall asleep in the tub with a book spread across my thighs.

She's trying to infect me with her ambitions, she talks about medicine, about chemistry, about astrophysics—she says that with a brain like mine, I could be an astronaut or work with minerals.

I made a calendar where I listed what to review each day: everything from the first year of high school to the last, from the Babylonians to Hitler, from the capital of Molise to the characteristics of DNA, from the aorist tense to Carducci. There can be no cracks in my knowledge, no leaks. I've got to be ready for anything.

At dusk, I'm like an owl, reciting Greek poetry by heart, practicing meter—iambic trimeter, dactylic hexameter, anapest. I try training my poor memory to become impermeable, built of steel and aluminum, to safeguard dates, kings and queens, rhymes and melodies, wars, epidemics, algebraic formulas, geometries, column capitals and paintings.

Iris calls sometimes, asking if I'm angry or if there's something troubling me.

I tell her no. I just need to study, study, study. She asks if she can be of any help. She invites me to meet up with her and Agata to review together but, stubbornly and coldly, I decline. I'm not turning back. Instead, I keep digging the trench between us.

Andrea says the maturità exams don't actually matter and that I'm letting myself get worked up over nothing. He's already in his second year of university, studying economics, with six exams under his belt. My mutterings are like a hungry kitten's meows to his ears. He lets me use his computer, but I keep my thesis topic a secret. I can't stand him being in the same room while I write, lounging with his phone, reading or listening to music. Even the sound of his breathing disturbs me, so I send him to the living room and lock his bedroom door behind him, turning the key twice.

He has to knock to be let back in. I open the door and he's carrying a plate of bread and prosciutto with a glass of pear juice. He sits beside me on the bed and says, Just relax. He keeps repeating *relax* as he twists my hair around his finger. I say I've already forgotten so much, I already can't remember three-quarters of what I've studied up until this point. I don't understand the end of history in Hegel. I don't understand—I don't understand what has ended.

He says I look very pretty dressed in white.

I blush, glancing down at the dress I'm wearing. Thin straps, full skirt—one of the dresses I like the least, but it was all I had left hanging in my closet. I've been studying too much, sweating through everything, changing outfits constantly. My mother hates me for this.

What does that have to do with anything? I say, tucking the skirt between my thighs.

We should go out dancing and you should put your hair up, he says, pulling my hair back with both hands, gently holding it in a high ponytail. He says that this way my face will be more visible.

I feel the heat on my cheeks and on my ears, which are now bare, exposed, gigantic and abnormal. I quickly cover them with my hands and tell him he has to stop.

Why? he asks. You look pretty. I like how you look.

I stay still as he combs the ponytail with his fingers. My hands remain over my ears. He looks at me, smiling, as if admiring a perfect circle.

Suddenly, I find myself back at that afternoon with the bumper cars when he wouldn't look at me and my feet were cold from all the emotion. Everything was spinning, everything revolved around him. I can feel him behind me as I lift the gun to shoot, I hit the target again and again and I win. There's no before or after, there's only that place—a hallway, a balcony, an underpass—where we're alone.

We can go dancing if you want, I say finally, taking my hands off my ears. He twists my hair into a bun, holding it in his hands like a bunch of tulips.

Andrea's body is thin, and when we're alone, in his bed and under the sheets, I lose track of north and south. I detach from my suffocating thoughts, from the endless blues, the dragons I battle—my teeth, my knees, my belly button. There's something about him that pulls me into the present and commands attention. I no longer hear the rustling in the hallway, the branches tapping against the window, the cars outside. When we're alone, Andrea speaks to me in a very soft voice and I can never quite catch what he's saying, but it's as if I already knew—as if I remember that lullaby.

The written portion of the maturità begins on Monday, but it's still Saturday night, and I let myself be convinced to go out dancing. Andrea insists because I'm wearing that dress he likes so much, so I close my notebooks, turn off the computer, and put my thesis away. I comb my hair, gathering it up on top of my head. He looks satisfied. I look like someone who doesn't exist.

We get take-out pizza and eat it sitting in his car. He turns on the radio and keeps changing stations, so I hear only bits and bites of songs. I wipe sauce off my face with the back of my hand.

The place where we're going is called Movida, it's a club below the Bracciano castle. Like most places on the lake's shores, it's only open in the summer. It has its own little beach with amenities: a volleyball court, a concrete dance floor, a small steel dock.

When we arrive, some people are there already, but it's not too crowded. It's Hawaii theme night, and someone hands us fake flower leis. I put mine on over my white dress, covering a tomato-sauce stain on my chest.

I follow Andrea to where his friends are sitting at the tables next to the dance floor. The music is deafening—eighties and nineties classics remixed sloppily, clashing with one another. The DJs yell clumsy prompts into the microphone, and their creativity leaves much to be desired. The songs—no matter how much the clubs change—are always the same. Over the months, over the years, over the decades, they've come to define us. They're the soundtrack of our region.

I say hello to the people I know, then wait for Andrea to get us drinks: a strawberry caipiroska for me, a Blue Angel for him. All around there's a jumble of faces from the towns nearby, people who always show up because there's not much else to do around here. The clubs don't even compete. There are only three of them: one for Thursday, one for Friday, one for Saturday. We orbit like satellites while they are our planets, our universe.

Iris sees me and comes straight over. She hugs me, stunned. She asks why I decided to come out and why I didn't tell her—I should have, we could've gotten ready together. I look like a perch caught on a hook, with my beach sandals on my feet and trigonometry formulas imprinted on my forehead—sine, cosine, tangent. Meanwhile, she has superlong lashes caked in mascara, flattering red lipstick, and a shorter dress than usual. I recognize it as Agata's. Sure enough, after a while, Agata appears too. They're dressed and made up almost identically, with only slight differences in shades and accessories. They look like they were cast from the same mold, mass-produced, sold in flashy boxes with embossed lettering.

I say we decided at the very last minute—Andrea wanted to pull me away from studying for just one night. They say how sweet that is, and how I look pretty with my hair tied back. Iris, in particular, fixates on this detail. She spends five minutes circling me, marveling at the length of my neck and the beauty of my nape. That's exactly what she says: You have a beautiful nape.

Have you written your thesis? Agata asks, playing with the ends of her hair, which she's straightened so perfectly it looks like gold and diamonds.

Yes, I respond.

What's it about? Iris asks. The two of us have never talked about my studies.

Cupid and Psyche—the myth, the statue, and lots of other things. I toss it out there without going into details.

But she presses, wanting to know which books I included, what citations I used, how I put my concept map together. She's acting like it's still the summer of reading and Batman and jumping off the pier. But it's not. It's a new summer, and she's standing tall in shiny heels while my head hurts, filled with thoughts of Schopenhauer, Apuleius, Canova, the way my Italian teacher chews her candy, and how she asked if I'd considered sending my CV to a supermarket—because yes, I have great grades, but let's face it: With a family like mine, now is the time to start working. Working, working, working.

Andrea comes back and says hi to them. I down my drink in just a few gulps, without even bothering to smile. More people crowd around us. Iris and Agata start dancing close, rubbing against each other, throwing flirty glances at the boys circling them. Ever since Agata broke up with the florist's son, she and Iris have been going out a lot. They make themselves desirable, playing with their clothes and expressions, but they hate being approached. They always dance together, entwined, in the middle of the dance floor, fishing for attention and leaving every desire for conquest unfulfilled.

I don't know how to do what they do. I don't seduce, I don't charm, I don't know how to sell myself—I never have. I watch them dance, smile at each other, drink. They keep inviting me to join, as if to say, You're one of us, you're wanted and well-liked. But I see the lies in their eyes. There's never been a place for me. I've never been in the right place.

Even Andrea tells me I should have fun, that's why we came, and he pulls me by the wrist and dances, moving his feet without rhythm, laughing at himself. He shouts that if he's going to try to dance, then I have to as well.

I feel like there's a noose around my neck—the open space of the garden, the fresh, humid air rising from the lake, the sound of ripples lapping the shore—everything is making me claustrophobic. I see myself inside a tin can, without any holes for breathing, being flattened by an industrial press.

Everyone around me is rotating their wrists and ankles, bumping into one another, passing plastic cups full of ice, letting black straws fall to the floor. Some glare at one another, some walk off holding hands, some kiss in the middle of the dance floor, brandishing their impudent, public love.

I shouldn't have come, I try to tell Andrea, but he can't hear me. He just keeps grinning.

And my friends sing, trying to be louder than the music. They shout and stare into each other's eyes, as if some electric current were passing between them. I'm incapable of tuning in to their frequency—that of people celebrating the end of high school, who aren't afraid of the future and who think they have a choice in the matter. They have houses, with or without mortgages; fathers, with or without ties around their necks; mothers who bake pies and watch quiz shows on TV; brothers who aren't in danger of going to jail, who get invited to their birthday parties.

The minutes tick by and more and more people arrive, forming one big, sweaty body—hair shiny with gel, shoes stained with grass. They pass cigarettes around, tossing butts and empty packs on the ground, letting their trash drift on the water's surface—all that waste they produce, as though it might just disappear, sink, and be forever forgotten.

One time Andrea told me I love you. We were sitting on the beach, competing to see who could count more falling stars, though it wasn't the best night for them. Not a single star fell. We were both left with nothing—no wishes to make. He'd finished off the bottle of red wine and then he said it. I coughed loudly, like I do at the dinner table whenever my father says he doesn't like the seasoning. I cleared my throat and feigned hoarseness, as though trying to cover up what felt like a miscalculation, a failure in the equation.

I tell him I want to leave, but Andrea insists that the night's just begun. He asks if something's wrong, says I can tell him anything, but I don't confess and I won't be absolved. I stay silent. My tied-back hair makes my scalp itch, and my breath feels shallow. I toss my empty cup in a trash can overflowing with other cups, other lives, and other thoughts. I don't know how to explain mine to him—he wouldn't understand. There would be no way to not appear ridiculous and mean in his eyes. How do you explain jealousy? How do you explain fear? How do you explain loss? How do you explain a future that will never come?

When Andrea gets distracted, chatting with a friend, I walk away. I move through the crowd, feeling the dampness of their bodies, the weight of their hopes against my skin.

There's no way to really leave. The Bracciano lakefront is disconnected from town. No shuttles, no buses. The only way to get here is by car or moped, and that's how you return home. But I don't care. I start walking on the side of the road, past double-parked cars, past groups of people lingering, deciding whether or not to go into the club. Some are puking up their dinners next to a poplar tree or a fake palm. Others toss used condoms on the beach.

I keep walking, past closed restaurants, shuttered pubs, white wooden stalls used for selling drinks and shaved ice during the day. My only company is the sound of the lake. It's not like the sea— there's no rhythm to it, no constant melody. The lake is usually silent, its water still and shiny, reflecting the night. Only the wind stirs it, making it sing, and even then, only briefly.

I feel like a white spot in the nothingness of a pitch-black night, out of place among all the colors and patterns. My hair is pulled back. I'm wearing my confirmation dress and those fake flowers around my neck. The tomato-sauce stain, the sweat under my armpits, my shoes going *flip-flop*.

Then a moped pulls up in front of me. Cristiano takes off his helmet, he tells me I'm crazy, it's late at night and I should not be out walking by myself, it's a bad habit.

I tell him it's none of his business and he shouldn't be following me.

He says he wasn't following me. He was going to pick up one of his friends in town when he saw me walking along the road, with my long legs and strange hairdo. He says I don't look like myself.

I look him over. He's wearing a shirt that's new but already crumpled at the collar. His cologne is strong, sweet, dizzying. His eyes are red—like he's smoked too much—and his shoes are untied. I'm happy to see him. Maybe that's how it works with the wrong people—you're always happy when you run into each other.

You know that guy I used to date—Luciano? Do you remember him? I say and take a step toward him. You robbed his house. Well, he texted me today, wishing me luck on the exams this Monday. On the phone I got with his money.

He laughs, which makes me laugh too.

I told you that guy's an idiot. We found a white teddy bear and the underwear he wore in kindergarten still in his closet, Cristiano says. He makes room for me on the saddle and hands me a helmet.

I climb on, struggling with my long, unwieldy skirt, and he takes off, fast as always, ravenous. He heads toward the main road, the one without streetlights, the one that skirts the water, the woods, and the campsites, that smells of pine needles and wild plants.

It's the road of our lives, the road we know by heart, the one where you can see the lake, distant but full, stretching from shore to shore—a darker spot in the darkness. It's the road with the Air Force Museum, with the swing club that was shut down in the seventies, with the plant nursery and its angel statues, the villas perched up high in the hills, and the foxes that dart out from the woods and under your car if you're not careful.

I grip him tightly around the waist—partly because I'm cold, partly because it just feels right.

After a while, he asks: Are you ready?

I know what he's asking, what I might be ready for, and I say yes.

Cristiano speeds up and turns off the headlights.

And just like that, we throw ourselves into the dark.

10

The Fire

1. The way you camouflaged, transmuted, transformed yourself into a copy of Agata, who, in my opinion, you'll never, ever, manage to resemble.

2. The irritating attempts you made to drag me along on nights out, for walks by the lake, and three-way conversations, even though I made it clear I wasn't interested.

3. The over-the-top effort you put into planning my eighteenth birthday, despite it being nothing even close to what I wanted.

4. The way you repeatedly brushed aside our friendship—ours, as in just the two of us, not ours to be shared with a third or fourth person.

5. That ridiculous poster with the word *courageous*, which I'd already told you has nothing to do with me. I folded it up and threw it into my closet—with all the other things I don't want to see every day.

6. The nights at the discoteca when I was excluded because I was dating Andrea and couldn't rub myself up against any male who happened to be passing by.

7. The phone calls that gradually became less frequent, then actually stopped entirely, as well as the nightly rings that were our code language, our secret. Above all else, I hold the disappearance of our secrets against you.

8. The attentive and friendly texts you sent while, in real life, things between us were cold and distant.

9. The fact that you didn't show up for my maturità, even though I told you not to come—I was hoping you'd break that rule. Then for yours, you invited Agata, too, and made your final dedication "To my friends." You lumped me in with her.

10. The idea that, just because of my background, you could turn our friendship into some kind of triangle. I hate triangles. I prefer straight lines: lines that connect two points and are always straight.

I wrote a list for Iris, like she asked, describing all the things she'd done to hurt me in recent years. I delivered it on my bike, to her house, and then weeks of silence followed.

Now I'm at Andrea's. It's afternoon and it's already dark outside. The houses in his neighborhood sit close together. They're painted orange and yellow, the gates are automatic, the edges of the hedges are shadows, and we're naked under the sheets of his bed, hiding. He says, Let's pretend we've disappeared together, like no one can find us.

Our breath is hot under the covers, our bodies are soft. My red hair is everywhere—in my mouth, under my arms, covering my eyes so I can't see. And yet I think that perhaps this small, cramped space—a bed, two bodies pressed together, our hips, our clavicles, our toes—would appeal to almost all the versions of me that exist, from the annoying to the aggressive, from the uptight to the arrogant, from the hopeless to the impolite.

I look at Andrea from this short distance and I'm drawn to his physical flaws. I look for them up close, like the mole he has on one of his nostrils; the scar on his lip; his pointy ears; the Adam's apple that has gotten bigger and now is noticeable when he swallows; the bones that stick out too much at times; the muscles that are underused and barely visible; the pallor that assails him even in the summer; his hands with their long, feminine fingers; the nails he often cuts too short; how he can't raise his voice even when he's mad; the blackheads he has on his back; the dry skin on his knees. I seek these small imperfections out, trying to come up with an explanation for why he's chosen to be here with me.

His bedroom has a queen-size bed and a small balcony. The shirts his mother ironed for him are laid out on the desk and the walls are light blue, the color of September skies. I peek around at his universe, breathing heavily and clutching my body to his as if to camouflage myself, to ensure I'm absorbed like buried sutures, the kind that close deep wounds. The body is forced to absorb them, incorporate them into its system.

My cell phone vibrates and I receive some texts, but I don't read them because I'm not there. We've disappeared, like Andrea said, and they can't find us, not even by shouting our names.

When I leave his house, my lips are swollen and my legs are warm. I look at my phone and see a message from Iris. She read my list and wants to apologize. She says she realizes now how much she hurt me. She's left her own list—the ten things she thinks are necessary for starting over—in my mailbox.

I stand still next to my bicycle, under a streetlamp with a flickering light, and I feel like I've finally got them both back with me again, like I've won them over, despite numerous raids and intrusions from others who tried everything possible to pull us apart.

My stomach is full of this confidence, this vanity. I get on the saddle and start pedaling home without touching the handlebars. I sing a song I heard on the radio. It goes: I'm back to square one, I'll turn off the lights and you'll be gone, for a few moments, beyond the fog, beyond the storm, there's a long, clear night—it will end, but it's the tenderness that scares us.

I enrolled in philosophy out of spite—to defy, curse, challenge. I enrolled with my diploma and my honors, with my now very long hair, my eyebrows bleached from summer, my narrow hips, and my practically nonexistent breasts. The part of me that needs to convince others of my worth led me here. They said certification course, medicine, surgery, office work—I said Martin Heidegger.

It would've been too easy to study languages, literature, or political science. I had to find myself a scourge, to go overboard, to search the sea for the fish with the most bones and eat it raw. Now I have the metallic taste of violent chewing in my mouth and the remnants of a bad meal stuck between my teeth. I don't know if I should spit it out in the grass or knock it back with a liter of aranciata.

On the phone I told Mariano: I'll study Marx and learn everything there is to know about capitalism.

He started laughing.

My studies are packed solid like a shipping container—windowless, boxed in, a spare structure no one will ever turn into a palazzo. I had to carve out new spaces to keep up my intellectual efforts, had to create new rituals and deadlines, rhythms and schedules.

I often find myself studying in my room, which never really evolved with me. Each year, it gets less lively, more impersonal. It looks like the bedroom of two children away on vacation. They left their basketball in a corner and their jellyfish- and starfish-patterned sheets all bunched up on their beds.

On the wall in front of my closet I taped up my class schedule, a list of books to study, a list of books to reread, a list of books to photocopy, a list of those already photocopied, a list of those I've found, a list of those I haven't found, a list of those I already hate, a list of those too long to be photocopied and therefore to consult in the library, a list of the illegible ones, a list of those I took my anger out on, a list of those with missing pages, a list of the missing pages themselves.

To study, memorize, understand, I have to write. There's no other way. I fill up notebooks and notepads with words, question marks, ellipses, half sentences, famous last names misspelled, arrows connecting dates and events, titles in quotation marks, quotations taken down in a hurry and smudged. In order to relate different concepts, I need silence around me, complete focus. I have to wring every last drop from my brain cells.

I split myself in two. One me is on the train, and the other me is on the platform. It's raining and the water is a raging river and the me on the platform takes cover as best she can under the leaky roof. The me on the train is passing by in that same moment, and for some reason the train skips this stop. The me on the platform just stands there and doesn't know how to get home, while the me on the train watches her through the rain-streaked window. Then two lightning bolts come down from the sky. One strikes the nose of the train and one strikes the tail. The me on the platform sees them hit the train at the very same time. What does the me on the train see? It's been a lifetime of the me on the train seeing things; she no longer knows what it would mean to not see the world pass by behind panes of glass, in that ordinary sequence of places she's never been, places familiar to her only in the way they appear and disappear.

As I think this through, a chorus of voices erupts from the living room—my mother and the twins rumbling and roaring, my father providing the countermelody with intermittent verses of his own, squawking. I can't figure out whether they're arguing or are just unbelievably happy. Probably arguing, since unbelievable happiness has never lived in our third-floor apartment.

I walk out of my room tense, both because they interrupted me and because studying physics as a philosophy student feels like some kind of joke. I didn't sign up for philosophy to deal with physics, much less a watered-down version of it—I walk out and shout: I'm studying Einstein's relativity, if you could please . . .

Then I'm struck dumb. There's an object on the kitchen table, a black object with a smooth screen, holes in the back for electrical cables and an antenna, and a button to turn it off and on.

Signora Festa wanted to throw it out, my mother says to try to justify its presence, its monstrousness, this surrender to the mundane that none of us ever saw coming.

My father rocks his chair back and forth, making it bang against the table, his thin little legs trembling from the impact. He's jittery and champing at the bit. What's happening in the kitchen will set the new rhythm of his life, it's the momentous change he never dared ask for and the blessing no saint had yet bestowed upon him.

The twins already have the remote in their hands. They're trying to figure out how it works. It's an old TV, must be at least five years old—garbage for other people, manna for us.

I say nothing and keep my distance from the table. It's not like I've never seen a TV before. I've seen plenty in other people's houses, in the windows of home-appliance stores, hanging up high inside pubs or bars. I've admired, hated, adored, forgotten about, and wanted many of them.

Not having a television was our misfortune and our peculiarity. It was something we could brag about: I don't have one, I have no idea what you're talking about.

For a long time, we found ourselves on the margins of discourse, and we breathlessly attempted to understand the meanings of other people's conversations when they had to do with something that was impossible for us to understand. Yes, we experienced the impossible, because either you have something or you don't. Either you can touch it, lick it, dust it, break it, or you can't. And for us, this not having was its own kind of foothold.

The ease with which my mother announces such a betrayal of her own rules, this encounter with the superfluous, with the unjust, confounds me. Like a doll with ringlets and lace on her skirt, I sit sweetly at the table while they fuss over the thing, my father's chair going *tock tock* against the wooden leg, and the kitchen feels like a black hole, sucking us all in. Its gravitational field provides us no escape.

After a bit of manual labor, a string of expletives, some shifting around of furniture in search of a hole to stick the antenna cable into, a reconfiguration of our needs, and the creation of an altar, the television is placed in the living room, against the wall and atop two fruit crates my mother usually reserves for potatoes and onions. She's already tying them together with wire, imagining how she'll decorate them with little flowers and PVA glue.

The twins get settled on the couch, eyes wide with excitement. My father finally frees himself from the table and heads over there, carefully positioning himself by first turning in a semicircle, and my mother sits on an armrest. The couch is small, it's not meant to accommodate all of us. We've never had any reason to all be in that room at once. Before, there was nothing to look at on the wall, and among us there was little to say.

The television is turned on and we tune in, lowering our immune defenses. I stay seated at the kitchen table, watching them through the open door, the backs of their four heads bobbing, their long necks stretching out. I can hear their comments; they've already started bickering. It's as if, by some tragic fate, their conflicting opinions end up reflected on the screen.

In no time, they're arguing about other people's arguments and they're arguing about whether or not it's useful to argue about this and they're arguing about the fact that after half an hour of TV they're already having arguments and they're arguing about the presence of the TV and they're arguing about the absence of the TV, about their unfamiliarity with national programming.

I stand up and no one notices. I'm hungry, but who knows when dinner will be ready. I go back to my room and stare at the paper where I'd drawn a train. I look at point A where the first lightning bolt strikes, and point B for the second lightning bolt, and then the arrow marking the movement of the train, and point M, which is me—me on the train, me on the platform. I know for certain that the me on the train is doomed because, if a moving train is struck by two lightning bolts at the same time, it surely won't make it to its destination.

One June afternoon, I go down to the lake with some books I need to study—the hermeneutic circle, Montaigne's skepticism, the trial of Galileo. I'm preparing for three or four final exams all at once, as well as midterms, practice tests, term papers. The breeze off the lake tastes like nothing, but I dip my feet in anyway.

The months of high school summers and splashing around, of long afternoons and lazy midday hours, are over. I'm trapped inside this new holiday, short and insufficient. Summer has become brief. By sunset, the lake looks like a tiger—the light splits into orange and black stripes, while night creeps in from the other side. Whenever I bring my books with me to sit on the beach near the borgo antico, I look up at the sky from the shore and watch the light disappear from the houses little by little. Even when there are no clouds, a haze thickens and conceals.

I turn to go back to my towel and see a girl just a few meters away. She's looking right at me and she has a small dog on a leash. The leash is blue, the girl is in yellow. She comes over, all smiles, and introduces herself: My name is Elena. I've seen her around before, from a distance. She always struck me as reserved, polite, with lots of friends. No one had ever introduced us, but I already know some things about her—what high school she went to, who her boyfriends were, and how, one night at Cigni, the discoteca in Viterbo, she got really drunk. While dancing, her little black dress slipped off her large chest, and more than one person swears they saw her left nipple.

I say my name back in a small voice. I have no interest in conversation. My head is wrapped up in my studies. The lake was supposed to be a companion, not a distraction. There aren't usually many swimmers in the middle of the week, even during the summer, and in the particular spot where we find ourselves, right by Pizzo Bend, there tend to be even fewer.

Elena says she knows who I am. She's seen me around with that girl who looks like an actress, and I say her name is Iris. And just like that, Elena sits down on my towel and lets her dog off leash. He trots off to sniff the rocks by the water. She starts talking, telling me all about herself. She says she wonders why no one ever introduced us, she's positive our paths have crossed before, and rattles off all these coincidences. She's studying to become a fashion journalist and doesn't know if she'll ever get good grades. She reads adventure books, likes to travel, and did ballet as a girl, but she has crooked feet and isn't very good at balancing.

I'm not interested in anything she's telling me. I want to pull out my books and pick up where I left off. I curse myself for having left the house. I should've locked myself in my room and put the fan right next to my desk.

Elena is overjoyed at our chance encounter, which I don't really understand or know what to do with. She seems kind, confident, and completely at ease. She cracks jokes. I think she's quite beautiful—her legs are tan but not very long, her breasts large, and her waist small. Up close, I realize her hair is dyed, and she tells me her mother is a hairdresser. She invites me to stop by her mom's salon, which is in front of the Church of San Francesco, but I tell her my mother cuts my hair—not as her profession but because we have no choice.

Elena suggests I stop by all the same. She could put semi-permanent polish on my nails as a gift—black, silver, gray (I look like the kind of girl who'd paint her nails gray), and then we could go get an aperitivo.

I say I don't know, we'll see. I'm not really into nail polish or sparkling wine.

We still exchange numbers before she leaves me to study. She stands up and brushes off her polka-dot dress with one hand and calls for her dog, Gin. Like gin tonic, she says with a smile. I watch her walk away, swaying her hips. Gin is on his leash once again and they are once again yellow and blue.

Ever since that day, Elena has texted me a lot. She's not pushy, she's not annoying, but she is persistent. She says she can come pick me up in her car—it's white and brand-new, like a city taxi—and that it would be nice to go to the sea, to Fregene. She also knows a private sailing club on the lake where no one ever goes and where the water is cleaner. They've got boats and a well-manicured lawn. She tells me about a recipe she found online and how she'd really like to try making homemade ketchup and dunking nachos and fries in it.

Her attention makes me feel valued, especially after all the years of Iris barely noticing me. So, without much hesitation, I start to join in on her plans. I find myself setting aside my books for several hours to head to the sea and drink margaritas on the beach. I pretend to know how to cook and improvise a guacamole. I watch TV with her father, a lawyer and bodybuilder, and her little brother, who loves the mountains and takes pictures of alpine ibex and wild goats.

Together we watch *Breakfast at Tiffany's* and *Sabrina*, her favorite movies. One night I sleep over in her bed, watched over by black-and-white fashion posters, clippings of Cindy Crawford and Naomi Campbell, and images of the New York skyline covering her walls. Her dream is to live in Manhattan one day, and also in California and Hollywood—anywhere with a view of the water. She tells me that in the USA, moli are called piers and they're superlong, not like our pier, which is short and slimy and useless. In America, people living near piers have amusement parks and the beaches are so wide you can play tennis on them.

While we're lying on striped sun loungers at that sailing club, sipping aranciata, I finally tell her something about me—about my stuffy, unhealthy house that seems to swallow up everything and everyone—a murderous house. I talk about my mother and father, about the absence of my brother, about the pink bear that Iris nicknamed Babol, just like the brand of gum we used to chew as kids, and about the twins and their incurable generosity.

I manage to string together some coherent thoughts and opinions on Andrea. I vaguely complain about our past but speak highly of the present. For the first time, I try to process everything I've experienced out loud, though I don't mention my nights of no-headlights with Cristiano. I skirt around certain events, trying to make myself sound interesting and mysterious. I repeat, Ah, if you only knew and Don't worry about it, sometimes I really do lose my mind, my mind is crazy. Suddenly it feels fitting and right that I would be part bad girl, part girl with the cryptic eyes—it makes me provocative, difficult.

I tell her that I, too, would like to live in some faraway place—the Congo or Japan or Polynesia—and I, too, wouldn't mind having breakfast outside a jewelry store every morning, just to sit in front of the window and contemplate all the necklaces and earrings I will never have.

Spending time with Elena feels so intimate and natural. It's as if we've known each other forever, as if she's always been there. When I'm with her, things I once thought unlikely begin to happen. Elena always finds a way to have fun while spending next to nothing. She never complains when I have to bring my books along to study, and she's already established some traditions for us—like driving to watch the sun set over the lake whenever we come back from the sea. The lake's sunset is subtle; the sun doesn't plunge into the water—the water simply reflects its dying rays.

We say: Ciao sun, farewell sun, and burst into laughter.

Iris isn't happy about my new friendship. She keeps telling me not to trust Elena and I feel like she's saying it out of jealousy and regret. Now that she no longer sees me alone or as the third wheel, she's afraid I might prefer someone else to her. This new power—the ability to spite her and starve her hope—thrills me. The world keeps spinning, you reap what you sow, both the good and the bad.

Elena doesn't have a boyfriend. She recently got out of a long-term relationship, of almost six years, and she wants to tell me everything about Alessio, her past love—from the color of his hair to how many times he dried himself off with the sheets after sex. So I talk about bodies, breakups, and love affairs, too. It's surprisingly easy. All I have to do is loosen up.

The exam period passes and I manage to not fall behind. I got two A+'s, one A, and one B+, which made me cry. I destroyed two notebooks and thought about chewing up four packets of photocopies— I'd studied and worked so hard, like an owl, a marten, like an animal who roams around all night and is simply trying to survive.

Elena took only one final exam and seems delighted that she can enjoy the next few months without a care. She convinces me to celebrate with her and tells me to invite Andrea and a few of his friends. I accept, determined to put my studies and notebooks aside for at least a month. And just like that, a new summer crew is formed, seemingly out of nowhere. Who knows when it'll fizzle out—it's a new comet.

To show off my newfound friendship, I also invite Iris to the festivities, and we all meet up in front of a beach club after they've folded up the loungers and pulled in the umbrellas for the night. We have three bottles of warm white wine and some music blaring from the speakers of a car with its windows rolled down. I drink and drink and drink, laughing, leaning on Elena, exaggerating every affectionate gesture, dragging her to go swimming with me. Andrea jumps in, too, and the others follow him. Iris stays on the shore, her hair dry, her face long, she's like a crow.

Her sadness makes me euphoric. I leap into the water and let my hair down, shaking it out. I have toned thighs and tiny calves, I'm pale, and my red mane looks like a bloodstain against the sky. I have all this unexpected beauty flowing through my arteries, the joy of having gotten what I wanted without even having to contort myself, without beating anyone up, without pushing and shoving—now I have something to brag about: the certainty that I am well-liked. Anyone who looks at me really does like me.

I laugh blissfully and tipsily, climb into Andrea's arms, and kiss him in the water. He's like a serpent and I'm an octopus. The music is faint but it rings in the air, and when people pass by on their mopeds, they honk, as if to say we're doing it right, we're cool and free and mature.

This is how I feel: like a ball of dough that has risen under a cloth, puffed up with air. I'm bloated and boastful of my achievements. My exams are over, Andrea loves me (of course he loves me), Iris regrets her "courageous" comment and the ten reasons she gave me to hate her, and Elena is a runaway bullet, heading straight toward the future. It's now clear that I can act any way and be anything I want.

I make a throaty cry, like some lake bird's call. I mimic the appearance of a protected species, moving like an eel. I pretend I have the webbed feet of a seagull, holding my breath as I do flips underwater. I had to struggle and destroy to get here, but now here I am: I, too, am deserving of happiness.

I drink a gulp of water from the lake and feel like smiling. It's sweet, sugary—this water, this swamp. It tastes like cherries, like clementine jam, like marshmallows. The lake's water is always sweet! I shout at the top of my lungs.

Again: The lake's water is always sweet!

I shout it at the top of my lungs.

⌒

Cristia', I need a favor. I need you to come pick me up. Bring two full-face helmets and two cans of gas. Cover your license plate.

I hang up and my hand's shaking. If I were holding a cup of coffee, I'd spill it all over the floor. I'm in my underwear and my breath is shallow. I look down at my feet—they're shaking, too, vibrating. I grab a black, lacy bra, clasp it over my stomach and turn it around, arrange the cups, then squeeze my breasts and adjust the straps. I step into the black jeans that had been draped over the chair and pull on my sneakers. I look around for a sweatshirt, but I'm seeing double, seeing triple.

It's been five hours and yet I've found no peace. It's impossible for me to sit down or lean against the wall. I've already peed ten times and lost fluids I didn't even have. I'm melting away.

The call came while I was eating an apple in my pajamas—I was peeling it expertly, holding the knife in such a way that I wouldn't hurt myself, and I removed the fruit's skin without taking my eyes off it.

Someone on the other end laughed, but I didn't recognize the laugh or the voice. They told me Andrea had done something. Did I want to know what?

I said no and hung up. Unknown number. Shortly after, I got a text from Andrea that read: *Forgive me, please, nothing happened, I promise, I'd just gone over for a coffee.*

I stared and stared at my Motorola—the old, the honest, the indestructible—and willed it to explode, with all its texts and contacts, with all the traces of recent months and weeks.

They called me again from a private number and I picked up: Your boyfriend is with your friend. We're outside her house. He's inside, and we've already rung the doorbell three times but he won't come out.

I shook my head from side to side, trying to shake off the impossible. They laughed—laughing, laughing, laughing at me—then hung up.

I called Andrea but he didn't pick up, I called a second time and he didn't pick up, I called three four five times and he still didn't pick up. So I scrolled through my contacts and called Iris.

Is Andrea with you? I asked her straightaway.

With me? No, I'm at my grandma's in Monterosi. Why? What's happening?

They're saying Andrea's at my friend's house.

It's not me.

In the background I heard the sounds of a kitchen, the TV, the regional news, dishes clinking in the sink, and I hung up.

I felt like I was being strangled, stabbed in the throat. I was on the verge of losing my senses and sensibility—I started pacing around my room, back and forth. I opened the window—cars were driving by on the street, dogs were out on leashes for their evening walks, I could see the tree that Bear had once helped me break a branch from.

I tried calling Andrea again and he picked up, sounding flustered. He babbled some nonsense—regrets, excuses, belated admissions. He said it had been an accident, that the two of them talked but just as friends, and he didn't know why someone had followed him there that evening. He'd only wanted to chat.

I have no idea what you're talking about, I said.

He repeated that Elena's house was free that night and they'd met up to talk, then something had changed, but he wanted to be the one to tell me about it. He knew it wasn't okay and now he's desperate—that's what he said, desperate—and that's when I seemed to wake up, opening my eyes wide to the room around me and to myself, and disconnected my phone.

Now I'm opening my closet door and sticking my hands down into the jumble and junk, the tattered clothes, mismatched socks, rulers, drafting triangles, worn-out notebooks, a tennis racket, the poster from my eighteenth birthday. Finally, I find it. I grab it and yank it out.

I shake out the Superman T-shirt—one, two, three times—then pull it over my head and slip my arms through the sleeves. I find my black sweatshirt, zip it all the way up, and pull the hood over my hair.

I tell my mother I'm going out and she says I'm always going out and it's too much and that tonight I won't be going anywhere. But at that point I'm already down the stairs and out on the street.

She no longer knows how to convince me with subtraction—she doesn't have the power to take anything from me. She can't tie my hands behind my back when I use them poorly. She can't take away my plate at dinner when I don't obey. She can't leave my underwear dirty when I come home late at night, because I've done everything she's ever asked—I stayed with her and I studied, I studied until I dropped. I want to shout back at her: Those days are over, Ma', when you had a say in whether I went out or not, when you sat by the door while Mariano and I ran around in the concrete courtyard, where there were no longer any syringes, where you'd killed off all the roaches and diseases. I'm mutating like a snake in the sun. I shed innocence like dead skin, while she looks the same as always, carved in the marble of her maternity.

Cristiano has a helmet around his elbow and two gas cans balanced on the moped's platform. I walk over and take the helmet from him, put it on, and pull down the visor.

He doesn't even have to ask what's going on: The whole town already knows. He doesn't question my rage because he understands it. That's why I called him—he knows what is just.

I take one of the cans he filled up at the gas station and, once I've climbed onto the moped behind him, I hold it between us. With this precious cargo in my arms and between his legs, we take off. I shout out which way he should go and he follows my directions, driving like we're racing against a ticking clock only the two of us can hear.

The street is deserted, it's long past dinnertime, and all that's outside Andrea Coletta's two-family home are parked cars, so I dismount, and I see his, with its AZ plates, radio antenna, greenish seats—this car is different from his father's (the one I unleashed my anger on the first time). This time, his is the one waiting for me, his personal vehicle with his favorite stereo and the air-conditioning he loves. Cristiano parks his moped on the corner and watches the shadows under the streetlamps. We still have our helmets on and are each holding a gas can. We grip them with gusto, and he looks over at me as if to ask whether I'm certain, whether he should proceed. I nod vigorously, moving my helmet up and down, so we begin our pas de deux, the main act, the coup de théâtre.

I open my can by removing the black plug and I leer at the shapes and sizes of the cars surrounding me, the detestable masses—I get closer and pour gas over the tires and the hood, as if they were my enemy's legs, arms, and spine. Cristiano's about to join me but I point in the direction of the other cars lined up—there are at least five in a row. He nods, he thinks it's a great idea. One car causes a stir, five spreads panic and fear—so he goes for it. We douse all five, soaking them better than ladyfingers for tiramisu, better than sponges in the shower—windshields, wipers, headlights, windows.

I'm breathing heavily in my helmet, choking back my anger. The anger I'd kept buried deep, that I masked during big occasions and watched dancing from a distance. The anger the world forbade me, though it's a part of me, and I want to cultivate it. My neck feels weighed down, my hands hot, achy. We toss the empty containers between the cars and Cristiano pulls a box of matches from his pocket. They're long and have blue tips. He lights five and passes me three.

I watch the flaming tips. They burn down before my eyes and I remember that New Year's Eve text—*I've been thinking about you*—and You look pretty in white and We're not really here, no one can find us under here. I remember the smell of his sheets, of his aftershave, of the condoms on the bedside table, and the towel around my waist, the shower door opening, Andrea walking out, Carlotta saying, Here I am, and I'm standing there soaked, I'm dripping with water, sweat, loneliness.

I toss one match at a time onto the cars and the gas catches fire, the smoke billowing fast.

Cristiano says we should leave and climbs back on his moped. He yells out in dialect, We have to go!

But I'm frozen, mesmerized by the sight of the burning cars. All destruction captivates me—it's like something from a fairy tale, watching things unravel this way, break down, fall apart. This is my new superpower: watching objects, houses, people while they suffer.

My eyes are open and full of guilt as I pedal along the asphalt curves, passing the walls of what was once a volcano—our lake, in fact, was born from an implosion long ago. The sun has gone down and I don't have a light on my bicycle. The street isn't well lit, so I rely on my memory and on the lights outside the houses. I don't signal to the right with my arm, I just turn onto the road heading to the Muses lakefront, where the discotecas and beach clubs are. It's the same section of the lake where I spent that first summer with Iris, where I met Cristiano, and where we celebrated the end of exams a few months ago, when I was drunk and thought everything awaiting me was filled with wonder.

I turn right again at the end of the road, where it's no longer paved, and there's just one beach club there, already closed. I can make out a wooden structure on the jet-black sand—the lifeguard tower, unusable because the wood is rotting. Climbing on it would mean risking its collapse. I spot her car, white like a taxi, so I pull over and toss my bike against the fence of the bar that now has its shutters pulled down.

Elena is sitting on the beach, illuminated by the glimmer of the moon and a dim streetlamp. There's no one else nearby.

I'd received a long text from her a few hours earlier in which she recounted the drama of her broken heart and the struggle against her own will and a series of other half-baked excuses. She suggested a time and place to meet, begging me to come see her one last time, claiming that only in person would she be able to explain. The punctuation was all messed up: there were random capital letters, accents instead of apostrophes, and *k*'s where there should have been *ch*'s. The sloppiness aggravated me to my core, deep inside my bones. She hadn't even taken the time to read over what she wrote, she just spewed out her sad excuses, her pathetic mouse squeaks, without a shred of dignity—without the respect that words, at the very least, deserve.

246 · GIULIA CAMINITO

When she sees me, she stands up quickly. She looks bewildered, like she doesn't recognize the person coming toward her in long strides, sneakers sinking into the sand.

Elena has an air of penance about her and her innocent eyes are wide. She swears that their mistake wasn't planned and that it just happened—like days happen, like flowerpots on the balcony, butterflies in gutters, pits in peaches happen. This was just one slipup among many on this overpopulated, exhausted planet.

She says it was an awful week for her. She cried every night, all night long (I hadn't cried at all, not even for one night, or half, or a quarter of one). And then there was that whole catastrophe on Andrea's street. Even the trees in the yards had caught fire. Thick black smoke was still rising from the burned-out cars the next morning. The tuff-stone walls were smoked and all the windows were shattered; his street now looks like a cemetery of sheet metal. Everything smells like burnt fabric, plastic, resin.

I nod as if I understand the extent of the misfortune, which has surely caused damage and turmoil and hardship, and the thought pleases me, it comforts me, because it wasn't a gesture intended to forgive, to relieve, or to spread kindness—I delight in what's left of this scorched earth.

Both stories started at almost the same time, like poisons injected one after the other: first Andrea's betrayal, then the blaze at Residenza Claudia, where the houses sit right next to one another and the yards have just enough space for bougainvilleas and olive trees. People aren't talking about anything else these days. They flip back and forth between hypotheses and conjectures. They wade through the muck of this pond without crickets or frogs, competing to see who can figure it out first, who has more news to share with the rest of the commoners: We're a carcass on the ground, and they're the dogs. They want fresh meat. They've begun gnawing on us from the tips of our elbows.

Elena doesn't have the courage to ask if I was the one who did it because she doesn't have the capacity to understand how or why I would have. She can't piece together the puzzle of my moods, of my neurotic moments, of my wild but calculated reactions, so she makes the situation worse and starts talking about us.

She tells me she really likes Andrea, she's in love with him and she wants me to understand the strength of that love. Without this understanding, her one-eighty wouldn't make any sense, it would just look like a bit of mischief, a thoughtless act. But when love is involved, what can you say? When you're in love, every action is justified, meaningful. Every action is poetry.

Their long acquaintance (which began not even two months ago) burrowed its way deep inside her, down into her guts, planting seeds of mutual belonging, and she couldn't bear to hold herself back from answering the call of her feelings. I wasn't sure that was exactly what she said, so I ask her.

The call of what?

Of feelings.

I nod yes yes, exaggerating the motion, participating in her confession with my whole body.

Years ago, Cristiano told me a story about our lake: Once, in the middle of the lake, there was a city called Sabazia. It was a prosperous place where trade thrived, the surrounding lands saw no drought or danger, and food was plentiful. But the people were bitter and malicious and no one possessed any redeeming qualities. So the city and its people were punished by God, who sent so much rain to pour down on all the houses, the city walls, the courtyards, the laundry hanging on the lines, flooding the farmyards, the pigpens, and the horse stalls. The water kept coming down and down until Sabazia disappeared. Only one maiden was spared, saved by a mysterious young man who had urged her to run away with him. She begged for God's forgiveness and took shelter in a distant church, where she swore to live a pious and saintly life.

I look out at the lake. It once again appears bleak to my eyes, motionless—it makes no sound and seems to be dying, fallen into an unnatural sleep.

I've lost track of what Elena's saying. She's crying now, dabbing her eyelashes with a tissue she pulled from her pocket. I hear her say that I'm vital and dear to her and that she didn't mean for any of this to happen.

It just happened, I say as though to show that I understand, I'm listening, I'm here.

She nods, looks at me, and responds: Exactly. As if the whole thing were a trivial matter. Everything seems to come back around, everything has a beginning and an end.

It suddenly hits me with absolute clarity: There is no city called Sabazia in the middle of the lake, just as there is no nativity scene under the pier. There are no ghosts in the Odescalchi Castle, no witches who wander the sand dunes after the sun sets—these towns live by their lies, creating myths about the rocks and volcanic stones, telling stories to exorcise the brutes and the shameless, punish them, wash away their sins. But stories aren't enough. They don't tell the whole truth, and it's clear to me now that there was no conversion, there was no surviving woman, no blessed woman—there are only fiery women, like me.

Then Elena starts speaking about our friendship, because it exists, it's alive, without a doubt. She says she recognizes something of herself in me. We found each other, and to walk away now would be like making an unnecessary cut with a scalpel. What would we do without this understanding, this double-rope bond between us? Why let a single moment, a simple mistake, ruin it all?

I'm reminded of something Iris and Agata wrote on the poster for my eighteenth birthday: *Friendship is born at the moment when one person says to another: What? You too? I thought I was the only one.*

This is when I move closer and kick her in the kneecap with the full force of my foot—like a donkey's or a cow's hoof. She screams out and bends forward to grip her leg, which is surely in pain, searing pain, and then I grab onto her blonde hair with both my hands—I can see its dark roots and sun-bleached ends—and pull it like I'm hauling a bag off a dock, like she's factory waste meant to be dumped in the water. I drag her across the black sand, carving a groove in it with her body. Her germs, her saliva, smear the shoreline.

Elena tries to wriggle away, she kicks her feet, waves her hands, strikes me, and I take her blows without succumbing to them. I feel like a mass of reinforced concrete. I have no cracks or fissures—nothing can stop me. I keep dragging her: her D-cup breasts, her size-small hips, her butt that's perfect for Brazilian panties, her slightly too-big nose, her feet that were never quite good enough for ballet.

When we reach the water, I kick her a couple more times and then take her head, pushing it under the surface. I climb on top of her, holding her down, holding her still.

It's hard to keep her from getting air because she fights like a live fish that was recently hooked. She forces her head up and takes in a gulp of air, then goes back under, kicks, scratches, yells, cries, and her voice goes *glug-glug*. My shoes and jeans are wet up to my thighs and I keep moving deeper out into the water and I keep using my strength against her body, as if it were a pile of soapy laundry to be rinsed, as if working a tomato-sauce stain out of a white dress.

I think of the pizza boxes open across our legs. The crust is crispy, the sauce dripping everywhere, and Andrea says: Let's go dancing.

My mind is crazy. You have no idea what will happen if I really lose it, I tell myself, drawing power from this image of me as fearsome and fierce. I fight against the laughter from that phone call, the excuse of having a coffee together in the evening, the abruptness with which it was all ripped away from me—while I was peeling an apple. I think of the joy I felt and the way I believed in it, nurtured it, cared for it, fed it, the way I always described what Andrea and I had as important. But in the end, it was just a part of the infinite vanity of youth.

This life—the one I have between my knees, in my hands, like a bunch of grapes, like a flimsy book—has to end, because that's how the cycle of eras, of animals, of seasons works: everything has an end.

Elena is responding less and less effectively to my attack, to my homicide, and the bubbles in the water grow faint. Her spasms get smaller, her movements more subtle. There are only a few seconds left—time enough to say goodbye, to say I love you—before she'll be gone.

Then I hear two people talking on the beach, a man and a woman. The woman says it's fifty euros for everything and he says fifty euros is too much. They're getting closer, they're walking on the sand, and it won't take long before they see us—me crouching in the water, her submerged.

I'm forced to let go, to abandon my rage, and Elena lifts her head, her face discolored, lost. She has the wide eyes of someone suffocating inside a plastic bag. She gasps in the humid lake air and I bolt off toward the road and toward my bike. I don't look back and I imagine it won't be long until she starts screaming and follows me with her car and runs me over on the way home, or until she calls for help and police cars show up under Antonia's window.

The policeman who's her friend, the one with the Sicilian accent, will tell her: I warned you to keep an eye on that girl. Your daughter's going to end up in prison. She almost murdered someone. But what else would you expect from a red-haired woman raised in such a family?

11

The Moon Fell Tonight

In the beech grove, neither dirt nor grass can be seen, only dry leaves without gradients, a mantle of light and crunchy little leaves, the color of caramelized sugar or almonds. Cristiano says the Oriolo Romano beech grove is different from all the others because it grew at low altitude. He says beech groves are the most enduring places on Earth—they've stayed the same for millions of years, from right after the Ice Age to today, or maybe less. But even if it was less, I still observe those long, narrow trunks as if they were my ancestors. They look naked, like they have arms and hands and fingers, brushing against one another. I imagine them lighting fires in caves when no one's watching.

This is my graduation party and there will be no other parties because I've banned them.

Cristiano is walking out in front of me, dressed in the same tones as the undergrowth. He's wearing a dark woolen cap, a bright-orange vest, and a beard sprouts on his chin. He's taller than me, broad shouldered, and he keeps adjusting his pants while walking as if they were falling down, even though they're not—he's wearing a belt. I can't see his small, close-set eyes, the pupils that always seem to be either too wide or too narrow. I never know if they're reacting to the light or the dark, if they're synthetic, if they've been drawn on with a dark-colored marker.

You should've worn something colorful, he tells me and keeps walking.

I have red hair. That's enough color. No one will mistake me for a rabbit, I say, following behind him.

I bet you won't do anything with your degree, not a thing, he says, his shotgun dangling beside him, next to his thigh and down to his knee.

I'll apply for a doctorate. I'm already working on my proposal. They'll accept me, and I'll just keep studying, I say confidently, gripping the shotgun he gave me—I look around, searching for low movements, dark spots, listening for animal sounds.

It's clear to me that this is what will happen. All I know is studying and memorizing and archiving. They have to let me continue. It's my rightful place in society. I'm meant to become a researcher or a professor's assistant, hang in there even though they'll pay me next to nothing, then take the national associate-professorship exam and become a university professor, write tomes, become a clickable link, a searchable entry in some faculty directory.

They even kill wolves with this thing, Cristiano told me about his lupara shotgun—he took it upon himself to tell me all the stories about his lupara and about mine, and about all luparas, the genealogy of the lupara.

I thought about how I wish there were wolves in the beech grove so we could experience a true hunt, a hunt for something vicious, something harmful, something that could devour us, whose shadow sleeps in the pit of every little girl's stomach—but instead I'll have to settle for thrushes and wild boar, creatures without fairy-tale nobility.

Hunting in the beech grove is prohibited, and either way, neither Cristiano nor I have a hunting license, but he knows the best hours and the areas where the game wardens don't often go. He knows how much time it takes to carry an animal carcass from the middle of the woods to his truck.

We don't have any dogs with us because they make too much of a racket and attract attention, so our hunt is slow and ill-fated. We have to wait for animals to move on their own or when they hear us coming. After what feels like hours of walking through the woods in silence, or else listening to Cristiano's tales about his grandfather and great-grandfather and about what happens in the shacks at the edge of the beech grove—the ones that look empty, but are in fact full of life, irrationality, misfortune—I see a wild boar, its pig head, its fat body.

It's standing next to a rock, rooting in the dirt. It would be too easy to shoot it like this, and there's no flavor in simple things, in cheap challenges, so I tell Cristiano to stand at the ready because something is about to come along. I raise my smoothbore lupara, take aim, and shoot a tree to get the boar on the run. It starts running, its short legs scraping the earth. Its bulk is a declaration of presence. It moves awkwardly through the trunks and the brushwood, it gallops across the dry leaves and grunts out all its worries. Cristiano shoots in its direction. He shoots twice and doesn't get it. The animal twists and turns in its escape, it sinks down low, searching for the guts, the spleen of the woods, the dark place where the shadows are ready to receive it.

C'mon, Cristia', get him! I shout.

He takes off in the direction of the animal and then stops and shoots again. He shoots and shoots and he doesn't get anything, and I think about how if it had been an angry wolf, he'd have already been mauled in the face, the throat, the chin. I move closer, then pass him. I search for the wild boar as though searching for myself.

I see myself on all fours in the woods, trying to escape the weight of my almost crimes, all the bad words, the angry gestures, the sweetness I didn't know how to give, the tenderness I wasn't able to receive, my future. I'm the one plodding along and crouching down low with my bristly, tough fur, an armor of leathery animality. I grunt, I sniff, I don't want to be stopped, to be put on trial or accused. I raise the shotgun, which to me is like a body, a living object. I take aim—one of the few things I know, and will always know, how to do.

I remember Mariano and me carrying Babol home by his head and his paws. We put him in our room and my brother starts laughing. I remember Andrea saying: Want to shoot? as he pulls some money out of his jeans pocket. He's talking to me.

I feel the shot going off and then the recoil. Thanks to Cristiano, I know that the lupara was used both by partisans and by mafiosi, by hunters and by fighters. The gun blast tears into the wild boar's flesh, and its screams are high-pitched. The shot is precise, like something you might see on the big screen, something that would be applauded and celebrated with a big, fancy party. The animal—tusks and hooves and muscles and tendons and all—collapses. Its thighs, stomach, and head jerk as it struggles to understand what hit it and how. It'll never know. And the end of its life is all there, in the not knowing.

I think about myself, about the end of my studies, about everything that I know awaits me, about everything that seems sure to happen, and about everything that I've never questioned. I've never had a summer job, unlike my friends. I never put any money aside to help me escape my mother's hovering. I only concentrated on my exams and my books. For years I followed the red thread between my fingers—for long months and long hours. When I lost sight of it, I longed for it. Now I'm outside the labyrinth, holding the Minotaur's head in one hand, looking around. I'm ready. I'm wearing my hero armor. Someone has to notice me. Someone will prepare a little corner of the world for me. They'll find a suitable place for my glory, my feats, and the duels I've won.

Fifteen minutes later, we're dragging the boar back to the truck. We're walking quickly—Cristiano with the front legs, me with the back, the legs tied with rope, the body suspended between us. We stop every so often. I would never be able to carry this weight without Cristiano, not even briefly, not even in a state of madness. He helps me, his face dark, knowing he failed, and I try to talk to him about stews and red wine and ragù and he nods, his eyes straight ahead and unmoving.

This was your gift, you can do whatever you want with it, he tells me, hoisting the animal onto the truck—its body makes a loud thud against the metal. Cristiano climbs up and covers the corpse with black plastic trash bags, he soaks up the dripping blood. My arms ache terribly.

He doesn't rush his movements. He carefully stores the shotguns and attends to the dead body and its liquids with a calm detachment.

It's his best quality, the sterile way he faces the world and its affronts. If something needs to be done, he does it. Cristiano is solid, certain, consistent. With a small inheritance from his grandmother, he bought a farm outside of town and is fixing it up. He spends his days repairing stalls, putting up fences, stuccoing walls. He was born in this place, and he is this place—he is his family, he is the lake. He's exactly as he seems, transparent, straightforward.

I'm the broken and opaque one, the one who refracts across surfaces and who is always only half seen.

Why the long face? You look like a dog kicked you.

My mother comes in and finds me leaning over the kitchen table, my eyes glazed, my lips like crumpled paper. She sets down the groceries, the potatoes, the artichokes, the skim milk. I rock back and forth with a foot up on the table leg, swaying.

No reason, I'm just nervous.

Did you talk to your professor about the doctorate? she asks, and I'm reminded of that man's long face, his little glasses perched on his round nose, his fingers constantly in his nostrils, rummaging, cleaning, pulling out, and starting all over again—digging deeper and deeper while talking, telling me my project is too literary, the figure of the idiot has been done to death, no one cares anymore. "How Do the Poorly Loved Speak?" is too fragile a title. We do serious research here and I can't even read German, so what did I expect? University isn't a courtyard for sad souls.

I talked to him.

What did he say?

He said that as the director he doesn't endorse his own students, in the interest of fairness, and that I should try at Tor Vergata, without a scholarship, I tell her. The open window lets in air that reminds me of the department's courtyard, where all hard work tumbles downstream, flies cover the walls in the summer, where everything is still and nothing can save you.

Without the money you can't do it, I've already told you that. What are they thinking? What are we supposed to live on while you're there, working for free?

Antonia uses her rallying tone—combative, insistent, like she's in the middle of a class struggle. She drops the artichokes into the sink, submerging them in water. The neighbors are listening to Latin American music and singing along. My father watches *Beautiful* while waiting for *Cento Vetrine* to start on Canale 5. The TV pumps its clean air into Massimo's lungs, necessary oxygen: all that blonde shiny hair, the shoulder pads, the miraculous resurrections, the uncovered betrayals, the overbearing mothers, the silences of love.

Don't start with me, Ma', don't start.

If I don't start, who will? All they're offering you are things that don't pay—and after all these years! We killed ourselves so you could study, with your grades, with all your knowledge, and now it's all worth nothing . . . Tor Vergata . . . I should go speak with that man myself.

I'm not twelve. I already spoke to him.

You didn't do it very well, not as you should have, otherwise he wouldn't have screwed us over like this—isn't he the boss there? And he tells you to go apply at some other university? If he can't take his past students, then who will? Who will take them? The Holy Spirit?

Whatever, I cut her off.

No, not whatever, you need to start preparing to teach in the schools then, find out how it's done, go ask them.

I didn't take all the required courses.

What does that mean?

I don't have enough credits in the subjects I'd need, like history.

How come?

Because I don't like history and I don't want to teach, Ma'.

Are you kidding me? Have you lost your mind? Antonia abandons the vegetables. The shopping bags are left open, the twins will be home from school soon, and they won't find lunch on the table. They'll wait quietly, whispering secrets in each other's ears meant for no one else.

I wouldn't trust myself with a child, not even during a war, I say, stomping my foot—one, two, three times. My foot goes *thump thump thump* and interrupts the rhythm of our argument.

If you didn't take the courses for teaching, what courses did you take? Why don't you take them now?

They cost two hundred euros each when you're not enrolled.

Then what are you going to do with your degree? What will you do?

Nothing.

Nothing? There's no such thing as nothing. Everything leads to something else. Find a way. Go to the office, go wherever you need to go, and stay there until you've fixed this.

I'm not going anywhere, I hate them all, I snap back. In my mind, I see the posted announcements, the seminars, the phone numbers for room rentals, the library's card catalog, the always-occupied computers, the classrooms arranged in semicircles, the easily jammed foldout desks, the soggy toilet paper rolls, the hum of the electrical box in the back, and I remember something that crazy kid Samuele once said, something I've never forgotten: The moon fell last night, the world's about to end. In other words: There's nothing to be done, it's over, they tricked us.

Marco, the Festas' son, was right—I should be worried about you. At first I laughed when he said that, but there's nothing to laugh about. What are you doing? What are you doing with your life, with yourself?

Who is Marco? Never heard of him, I say, though I know exactly who he is.

He was at my eighteenth birthday, in a striped shirt, his chin smudged with frosting from the cake. He wandered around the party somewhat tipsy with that frosting on his face. I am horrified and disgusted by his pale, lanky frame, and all his castoffs: the bicycle, the shirts, the pants requiring alterations, the board games with missing pieces, the five-year-old television. We've always lived off his leftovers. This is what I see when I look around our house: a junkyard of things the rich got bored with.

You've heard about him a thousand times, you've seen him just as many. You should really get to know him, I've been trying to tell you that for a while now. He's a good guy. He studies medicine.

I want to laugh out loud, to whistle with laughter, but I can't. I'm too tense and my belly feels so bloated I might as well be pregnant.

He's a fine young man, not like that Cristiano guy you're always hanging out with. He's a lunatic.

You know nothing about Cristiano.

You like him because he's cute? Look at me: I married the looker of the hour and you've seen how that turned out. He fell at his shit job and now I'll be carrying him to my grave.

262 · GIULIA CAMINITO

He's here, he can hear you, I hiss. He's my father, not a houseplant.

Massimo doesn't move his head or his ears. He doesn't change his posture: His eyes are glued to the screen, his pelvis pressed against the chair, his legs shorter by the day, like toothpicks. He's got the freshly shaved beard of a good-looking man who wears misshapen tracksuits and ancient socks. He's a beautiful larva, an optimal flowerpot.

Let him hear. He'd never do anything about it anyway. We're going to end up in the sewers.

I'll find something.

No, you won't find something, you'll find the job you studied for. You're not going to work at some florist or bar, or restaurant, getting paid under the table, without insurance, without vacation . . .

I already know this story.

You know it? It's not a story, it's our life.

Your life.

Your life is my life.

The silence that follows swallows me whole. What she said eats into me. I feel it chomp down on me. I have to react. I need to get away from her. My life is not hers, my life is mine, my life is my business. I build it and I destroy it—so I react, like a marionette swallowed by a whale along with some plankton, I jump and kick to get out and back into the sea. I surface, and I navigate by sight. I won't let her assertion or the sounds of her words eat at me. I look at her, furious, and jump up from the chair as if I'd been stung between my thighs. The prickling sensation moves higher, slipping into my underwear. I clench my buttocks and try to shake it away, but it's already in there, building a wasp's nest: the harsh awareness of our life, our condition, our roof, our dishes, our future, our investments, our groceries for lunch, our nonexistent money.

My life is not your life! I scream. I scream from deep within my bowels, from the younger me, and I feel the earth open up, the trees fall—there are mudslides and crashing thuds. My face is hot, my hair electric, my legs itch, and there's a creature inside of me, raging, despicable, fed up with being contained.

Massimo turns his head, very slowly, as though it were nearly impossible for him, and takes pity on the walls, the washing machine, the trash under the sink, the toilet that needs to be flushed as many as four times in a row to actually work, the laundry that fell down to the street, the detergent-bottle caps that we reuse as bobby pin holders, and maybe even me.

I leave the kitchen and leave my mother, who is as silent as I've ever seen her. My savage cry turned her mute. I storm into my room and lock the door.

Why is she always against me? She's like a dam that won't budge. Why doesn't she get closer to me, like mothers do? Or at least the kind of mother I want. She doesn't kiss me, she doesn't caress me, she doesn't brush my hair, she doesn't reassure me, she doesn't encourage me, she just judges and insists, she just humiliates me with her words and accusations, and she always brings up the end of my hopes and dreams.

She makes me feel inadequate, like a failure, a broken gear, a pendulum frozen at six o'clock in the morning when it's still the middle of the night. I feel out of sorts. I'm a misfit. I don't know where to turn, who to call on, or if I'll make do, because I don't know how to make do. I only know how to wait for my mother to make do on my behalf.

I think of the anise-flavored candies my Italian teacher used to suck on and her recommendations about getting a job, because that's what I should have been aiming for instead of wasting time and fumbling and imitating a life that is not mine, an untouchable career—how pitiable, what a poor thing. No scholarship, no support, no plan. All that's left is me, and I'm not worth much.

I look around my room and feel like I want to explode. I pull everything off the shelves and walls: all the notebooks, the photocopies, the books, the outlines, the summaries, the notes, the calendars, the dates, the deadlines, the forms, my name cut out and taped to the closet (a name that doesn't suit me, that I hate hearing said out loud), books about the universalism of difference, the rhetoric of recognition, biopolitics, messianism, secularization, the Leviathan, the second sex, the nomadic subject, skepticism, redemption, urban thresholds, the color spectrum, egocentric speech, sadism, Sartre's *Nausea*, Aristotle's *Metaphysics*. Everything ends up tossed in the air and splayed on the floor and I trample on it all.

Then I see it, straight and sturdy: my dictionary. It's sitting there serenely, fearing no judgment or malice, so I attack it. It was the first to mislead me, to make me believe I could change my life with words, that I could rewrite it, narrate it in first person. But no, it's always other people who tell our story and come up with our definitions, our brackets, the roots from which we are derived.

The dictionary is on the ground and I'm on top of it. I slam it against the floor as though hammering a nail. I wait for it to do something, to defend itself, but it doesn't have a voice and it gives in to my attack. Books suit me: they're defenseless and, as inert matter, they always submit.

Even *melologue* failed—we all know it. The universe doesn't seem to need it. It's in the cellar of obsolete terms like *helmsman* and *gaberdine*, *inkwell* and *gaiter*, alongside proverbs and heavy dialects, anecdotes and nicknames—all the things we've forgotten.

Babol is still sitting in his corner, but he's lost his luster and is an impenetrable witness to my banal fury, my disaster.

1. Teach me to jump off the pier with courage.

2. Try riding a horse and follow me into the woods.

3. Let's visit Batman's grave and sing him a stupid song.

4. Let's talk about our fears.

5. Let's write each other a letter.

6. Let's go back to Martignano and rent a pedal boat, then pedal across to the other side.

7. Let's go to Vicarello, because that's where the best sunsets are.

8. Let's argue out loud and get mad at each other.

9. Let's get back into the habit of ringing each other from our landlines when we get home safely at night.

10. Let's forgive each other.

I find Iris's list in my desk drawer, under the ID where I have a bratty look on my face, some expired caramel candies, a pack of pads without wings, and a pair of little scissors for cutting my nails. My room is a battleground between me and myself, between me and my mother and the house, between who I once was and what I've become. What species do I belong to now? Maybe I'm a lynx, an eel, a dinosaur. I come from the past and that's why the present feels so constrictive, like it doesn't have enough room for me.

Of Iris's ten commandments—meant as a truce, to ensure eternal peace—I respected none. I had many months and years to catch up, to make up for my mistakes, but I procrastinated. We could always do it another day, we could always watch the sunset the following evening. Any forgiveness could be left unspoken. No one would be draining the lake or uprooting the pier. Iris's rabbit had been dead for a while now and that's how he would stay: dead and buried in the back garden, between the lettuce and some eggplants.

Iris suffered my delays, my distractions and disappearances, but she kept inviting me over to her house to make muffins together, to watch a TV show about vampires, to walk around the vegetable garden. She offered to attend my thesis defense and invited me to hers (I declined both). She came to my house to show off the used car she bought after she learned to drive. She texted me late into the night and rang my house phone, but I didn't reply, I didn't pick up. She called so much that my mother started unplugging the phone and, as a result, it always gave a busy signal. Busy because, in fact, I was busy—busy digging deep trenches around myself.

All this time, I'd been wallowing in the most futile and fleeting conversations, never telling Iris about any of my fears, or my shame, or my difficulties. I didn't share anything about the fights with my mother, my struggles at school, the way Andrea left me feeling drained and emotionally numb. I didn't tell her about my low self-esteem, my callous urge to hurt and sink people as if they were fish, and I the hand clasped around their slippery bodies in the fountain of everyday life.

Iris has always kept the fantastic and valiant version of me in her emotional memory, the reliable and smiley me, the victim who doesn't dismember other people's bodies, someone who belts out songs in the car and reads books outside in the shade—a fleeting me, who lasted the length of a season, an evanescent image, a face underwater during a breath-holding competition.

When Iris found out about Elena and Andrea, she immediately took my side, fierce and warlike. She appointed herself as the messenger between me and my ex-boyfriend and delivered the final word to him: You're done. You're a period at the end of the last sentence. You're the conclusion.

Soon the whole town will find out what kind of people they really are, she'd say, comforting me with her certainty that there would be an altar and an executioner for them, that the axe would fall on their heads, breaking their white, chicken-like necks. I wondered: Where will their heads end up? Will I ever be able to start a collection? Now that all the books have disappeared from my shelves, I have space for my enemies' severed heads. I'll dust them, gaze at them, caress them—mocking and pitying them—all while knowing they've fallen thanks to me. The whole town will find out what kind of people they really are and their reputations will be lowered into boiling oil, left to fry for so long they'll no longer be palatable.

Iris never believed that I could've been the one who set fire to the cars in Residenza Claudia. For her, that idea was entirely inconceivable, it belonged to the realm of never going to happen. She didn't see me with my pants soaked up to my thighs, immersed in an attempted murder.

When the rumors ran through town, when the assault was reported, Iris stood behind the version of the story that protected me: Two girls had kicked, slapped, and punched each other over some boy. Just a simple case of lovesickness. And this telling of that night—new, improvised—caught on and led everyone to believe they'd just heard the obvious conclusion to a trivial farce, a dispute between teenagers, the kind of argument that, in three years, the two girls would laugh about. With time, everything that was once serious would seem light as a feather.

Iris knew I was innocent because it couldn't be otherwise and because Elena had already proven herself a liar. Between the two of us, she was the one who deserved to not be believed.

The whole town convicted and acquitted, whispered and followed the rumors that Cristiano had started. At the market and at the gambling house, on the lips of those who sat outside the bar in the piazza, of those walking arm in arm along the Soldati promenade: Two girls beat each other up, they used to be friends, but then the blonde slept with the redhead's boyfriend and the redhead got mad and the blonde did too and they got into a fistfight. The blonde can't be trusted; the redhead did the right thing. I would've beat that slut up, too, if it had been me.

Iris had nodded and said of course, that's exactly what happened. In her imagination, the scene unfolded under the moonlight: I was getting pinched and screamed at and my rival fell to the ground, and even there beneath me, she still hadn't paid enough for the harm she'd inflicted. She kept insulting me and looking for ways to make mincemeat of me—an assault within an assault, blame upon blame, conviction upon conviction.

Iris said she's keeping an eye on Elena Corsi's Facebook and that she'll always know who she's seeing and where. If a picture with Andrea ever pops up, we'll see it and retaliate, restart the rumors, circulate even worse ones—rumors that will cut deeper than knives ever could.

I told her okay, you do that, because I don't have any social media—the ability to look inside other people's lives like that terrifies me. It's like the eye of the webcam in Carlotta's bedroom that ransacks and spies and comments and shares our bare existences, the underwear we wear at night, our missing bedsheets, the folders on our desktops named LOVE.

Iris kept reassuring me that none of this was my fault, because I'd trusted her. I was the good one, the naive one, the martyr, and I would be rewarded for it. Blame goes around and comes around, goes around and comes around, goes around and comes around for whoever is guilty.

I reread her list and realize that these ten things are no longer the things Iris and I will do to repair our friendship. Instead, they're becoming the ten things we'll never do, the ten things I've lost, the ten things to mourn, and I feel like I'm back in the middle of the beech grove. My legs are stubby and hairy, my ears elongated, my nose like a pig's. I'm rooting about, my hooves are dirty from the woods and my stomach is filled with acorns, insects, larvae, eggs, berries, mushrooms. I sniff the air and then a shot goes off: someone has come to kill me.

Summer descends on the lake, bringing with it orange granitas, greasy potato chip fingers, beach umbrellas carried under arms, rows of sun loungers, ball games on the shoreline, and the hum of the firefighters' helicopter lowering some kind of giant bucket and gathering water to put out blazes. There are fires in the hills and pastures, sparking from the electrical boxes.

For the past three months, Iris has been shut up in her house and she only responds to text messages, not phone calls. She tells me she's watching cooking shows on TV—ones where they talk about farmed salmon, wild chicory, alpine cheeses—and in the mornings a nurse comes to give her an IV. She refuses to tell me why, or what the treatments are for, or what her illness is. For a while, I don't insist. Instead, I draft long and listless texts about my job search, about my mother who has stopped talking to me, about time passing and leading to no resolutions, no improvements. Birthdays, anniversaries, and holidays go by, and I'm even sending my CV to butcher shops because, you never know, maybe my degree will somehow help me weigh ox quarters.

The summary of my life takes up one page and that's it—I don't have any work experience, I don't have certifications, I don't have language skills. I've done nothing but study. I don't know how to explain to whoever reads my CV that the years I spent hunched over books were an act of self-denial and that I respected the social contract. The status quo is what kept me a student. I was never early or late with anything; I dutifully carried out the required steps of my education, and now that I'm educated, it's as if I've turned back into a mass with no dimension or depth—a useless agglomeration of knowledge—when what's expected of me is experience, which no one seems to be able to give me.

Summer knocks at the door with its heat and its lakeside lure. Piazzas and alleyways are crowded late into the night, bars extend their hours, wooden kiosks make coffee from the morning on, people who aren't rich enough to buy houses on the sea flock to our town on vacation from Rome, and the algae that crept up onto the shore during the winter has been cut back by the beach-club owners—the stones and the dead fish are gone. The lifeguards are back in their red T-shirts, certified at the same hotel pool where my friendship with Carlotta ended.

I ride my bike to Iris's house and ring the bell. Her mother answers through the intercom, telling me I can't come in. My friend is sleeping and they have a lot to do. It's best if I don't come back. She says Iris will call when she's feeling better. I tell her I brought a bag of lemons—my mother picked them from the Festas' tree. They're fragrant, perfect for seasoning fish, or you can use the zest in desserts. She says I can leave them there, they'll come down for them. I abandon my bag in the sun and ask myself why, of all the things I could've thought to bring, I chose something so sour.

The days go by and I decide to call Agata. My Motorola screen is cracked, a violet stain stretches across it—so I have to hold it at an angle to read text messages and telephone numbers, while everyone else I know has phone plans with internet and they're texting each other fifteen times a day. Agata picks up, surprised. I haven't called her in years. I've seen her less and less since the end of high school and we don't have much to talk about anymore. She works for her family's business, as expected. She's bought herself a Louis Vuitton bag and parades it around during the nights out on the pier, and she's always wearing artificial nails in colors like amaranth, turquoise, navy blue, adorned with rhinestones, with pearls, with butterfly wings.

Agata says she hasn't heard from Iris in a while. Their friendship has cooled over the years. Whenever Agata reaches out, Iris doesn't respond, and she even deleted her Facebook profile. One week she was there, the next it's like she's disappeared, she's retreated to the shadows and denied us access. I think it's her way of punishing us. We were too superficial, too full of vices. Neither of us stood by her side as we should have and now she's shut us out to teach us a lesson. I take the apparent calm of her silence as evidence. Nothing serious is happening; she's just stationary and sick, for now but not for much longer. Her illness will pass like clouds or storms, just as fog rolls away and frost melts.

After talking to Agata, I start thinking about the clues Iris left behind. I mull over the time she said she had a stomachache, the time she declined another slice of watermelon, when she said she had swollen legs and a hard belly, when she implied that she'd lost weight and her body was becoming so small it could fit in one hand. Yet none of this helps me picture her stretched out on her bed or on the couch, next to the remote control, far from the sun, from the stables, from the vegetable garden, from me.

I try to make up for the lost time, bombarding her with smiley faces and hearts—those awful less-than-three hearts. I make lists of activities for us to do once she's better and add them to the ten she came up with for us. The list grows to twenty, thirty, fifty-two things we can do when she's better, and I send them off to her in an endless stream of text messages, using up all my phone credit. She responds to this ill-fated list with a single smiley face.

It's this way of communicating at a distance—pressing keys and numbers, the symphony of a forced estrangement—that's the problem, so I start biking around town, to the bar, the fish market, the piazza, the clothing store my mother likes to go to. I interrogate the mannequins, the for-rent signs, the alleyways, the Collegiata church, the crusty statues on the corners of buildings, and the fountains spraying water and moss. I ask them what's happening to Iris, what's keeping her shut inside, because I'm sure the town already knows and they're plotting to keep me in the dark and make me suffer.

After a week, I go back to her house and the bag of lemons is still there; they've cooked in the sun, drowned in their own slime. There's a rancid smell and the stench of carrion. I take them and throw them in the dumpster.

Nonbelligerence and mutual indifference reigns at my house. I've become the dependent daughter who doesn't yield anything, doesn't multiply, doesn't cash in, doesn't cook, and doesn't have any riches or receive any handouts, the daughter who was never kicked out and who has never returned, the pillar of salt everyone is forced to see at dinnertime. And yet I'd like to ask my mother what I should do, since she's always coming up with solutions—how to get moving and figure things out. I've only ever taken up arms and attacked barricades. What she does is a project; what I do is war. In the first case, the purpose is clear; in the second, the only certainty is that it's best to destroy other people before they even have a chance to think about it.

I tried to talk with Mariano about Iris. I called him late one night after the moon had set, and he told me that there are people who don't want to show their physical pain, people who need to be alone when they're sick, and people who would hate for their illness to become a talking point. Like our uncle who, up until the day his heart burst, whenever he felt dizzy said it was just because of the sun, and instead of talking about himself he preferred topics such as horse racing, elm trees, highway construction. I told him that her silence made me angry and it wasn't because I wanted to be a witness to her disease or to publicize her fatigue. I just wanted to know what was going on. I just want to see her, see what her face looks like, give a name to things.

But the more the days pass, the more my brother seems to be right. Communication from Iris is sporadic. I write her morning, noon, and night, and I only receive a response to about every ten text messages, in which she usually says, *Yes thank you, all good, no thank you, see you soon.*

Then I get nervous and get on my bike. I hover—like a fly with leftovers—around her house, waiting for signals and movements. I wonder if she's broken a leg, or maybe she's burned her face, gone blind in one eye, took a blow to the head and now has a big scar on her scalp and short hair, has vitamin deficiencies or malabsorption, cramping from some form of early arthritis. Maybe she feels ugly and doesn't want her feeble, shameful condition on display.

But then I see her leaving the house. Her mother is behind the wheel of the car and she's in the passenger seat. She has short hair, her face is sunken and very pale, her shoulders are protruding, her neck is fleshy, her eyes seem to have grown big and dark, her forehead is wide, and her lips have deflated, they seem to almost fall off her face. The person I see through the windshield isn't her, but some stranger who's consumed her.

Iris! I say, and wave my hand without approaching, but they back up and drive away in the other direction, leaving me alone with that monstrous image.

Not much time passes before the entire town knows—doctors, nurses, people who've caught sight of her, her mother's friends, her father's excursion buddies. Someone opened their mouth and now there's nothing else to talk about. People concentrate obsessively on the why and the how, make assumptions, bring up blood tests and colonoscopies, whisper in bewilderment, cry, hang the damages and losses out on the balcony. Each of them contributes as they're able to the narrative of the new Iris, forgetting the old one, forgetting the Iris who was my only friend.

I saw you in the car the other day, you didn't look like yourself.

I text her and she doesn't reply, so I send the same message three times because I demand an answer, I need her to tell me: *That wasn't me, someone else is pretending to be me, I'm hiding out at these coordinates. I'll wait for you on this day, at this time. Don't be late because where I'm hiding isn't safe. Soon I'll be going somewhere else.*

The very same day I get a response from a perfume shop, Cristiano calls me. The shop tells me that, given my knowledge of philosophy, I could be a good fit for them, as they recently opened and are specializing in relaxation, body care, and yoga. Cristiano breathes heavily on the phone and cuts in and out, disrupted by an unstable connection.

Cristia', what's going on? I say over and over again, and I can only hear bits and pieces of what he's saying. Then all of a sudden his voice becomes clear.

She's dead, he says calmly.

Who? I ask because I don't understand and I'm steadfast in my incomprehension. I don't want to be open to an explanation.

Iris. I'm sorry. Her uncle ran into my dad at the business.

It's not true. He lied.

No, she was very sick. They brought her to the hospital a week ago for pain treatment. Her mother tore the room apart. There won't be a funeral. She's waiting to be cremated.

Who?

Iris.

I tell him he's lying and that I'm sick of his stories, his tall tales, his inventing names and facts, his babbling on. I hang up. Iris is not waiting for anything. Iris is home and now I'll text her and she'll respond, and that's what I do: I write her text after text and her phone gives me no response.

I dream of her that night. She's sitting on the edge of a house in ruins, on the third floor. She says she's waiting there. It's not like the world has ended. The moon is still in the sky.

The next day, they paste up the death-announcement posters. They're different from the others. There's a photograph of her face, and underneath, her birth date and death date. She's been dead for three days and now this is how the world is telling me, at the corner of the Viale Poggio dei Pini intersection, on an iron surface. Her death is on top of the other deaths. It will catch the rain, it will catch the cold, it will wear away. Her death will be covered up with the poster for the local fish festival. It's summer, and everyone is looking forward to frying up some lake lattarini.

12

The Taste of Gasoline

I ris and I saw a plane fall from the sky—or rather, a helicopter.

We were sitting on the beach and sharing a towel. Our bathing suits were wet, our shoulders covered by our dripping hair. We watched the lifeguards coming in and out of the water, out and in. Iris had her sunglasses resting on top of her head and she was licking a strawberry Popsicle. I had sandy hands and couldn't stand the children's screams, the way they'd been raised outdoors, coddled, reassured, made to shout.

Bear had wrapped Marta's towel around his head like a turban and was strutting along the shoreline, followed by Ramona on her tiptoes, telling him: Do a little dance.

Marta had brought a disposable camera. She started photographing them in yoga, top-model, and contortionist poses, like circus acts.

I could hear them laughing and jumping around, competing to see who could avoid burning their feet on the hot sand.

The Greco had gone to get some water and sandwiches at the bar. He came back with his fuzzy ankles and that hair of his, shiny as plastic, glued to his forehead. He offered us a tramezzino and a can of Sprite, which we shared. Iris drank from the right side, I drank from the left, one sip each, fizzy bubbles on the roof of our mouths, under the blazing sun.

The Greco sat down next to our towel, beside Iris, and very subtly tried to make some space for himself, to gain a corner of fabric and get closer to her. It felt like he was on top of us, like a horsefly, and I told him that Bear was calling him over, told him to go and take some pictures with them, that we'd print them out later and hang them on the wall. Even Iris told him: Go on, go over there.

He got up and scurried away, casting wistful glances back at us. We smiled at each other and Iris said: He's always rubbing up against my thigh.

Then a noise rose from the lake. A helicopter appeared from the inlet, black and compact, like a hornet. It buzzed and buzzed, putting on a show. It was swerving, rising and falling, moving its tail, doing a crazy dance, and people clapped, thinking it was a show, a surprise meant to entertain the lifeguards.

The aircraft leaned to the side and then tried to straighten out, only to tilt again, precariously on one side. We were all watching, thinking it had to be planned—surely it was some drill from the Air Force Museum or one of the many beach clubs with two-seater aircrafts.

Then, amid the laughter and wide-eyed children, the crash: The helicopter touched the water and overturned. It exploded. In less than a second, it went *boom*.

A blaze, a cloud of smoke, the propellers and nose submerged. From the public beaches came screams, and the lifeguards were already in the water, rowing paddleboats with their strong arms and low-cut tank tops. From the sailing clubs, they set out in motorless boats toward the wreckage. From the beach clubs, there was a fearful silence.

Iris had jumped to her feet, screaming: Somebody has to save him!

And I'd taken the towel, the can of Sprite, the last bite of the tramezzino, and dragged it all away. This wasn't our problem to fix.

Some people are simply doomed, I thought. We never found out who—by mistake, for fun, or due to bad luck—had vanished in the water that day, gone up in smoke.

The team of divers never found the body, just scrap metal that the boats dragged in. The lake wasn't swimmable for days after. The stench of gasoline lingered on the water's surface.

⁓

Dear Iris,

They've always said it's clear from my writing that something is tormenting me, and now what's tormenting me is you.

It torments me to think about your shoes with the heels and the fringe and the shiny boots and the sandals with the rhinestones, all in a row under the window in your room, about your fingers on the remote control while you search for a cooking show where a man with a potbelly and a nice face talks about cheeses and goats, about you wobbling your head to imitate the Trevignano bar guy, because he has too much hair and it looks like his brain is weighing down his neck, about how that head wobbling turned into something else over the years, a code, a way to say, Let's go to that bar, even though by that point they'd fired him, about how you looked underwater, your trembling outline and the shadow of your face, about your feet that you claimed were always swollen, about the way you'd say, This is no way to live, and would start laughing, about the things you gave new names to, about your fears of deep water, fires, lies, about that New Year's Eve with the florist's son and the face you made when I left, as if to say, Why are you abandoning me?, about having left you there with people you hardly knew and a scarecrow in flames, about having asked your grandma to knit scarves and sweaters for my entire family without ever even thanking her, about when I'd come over to your house and she'd be sitting behind a curtain on the first floor and she'd smile at me, about the hospital and about the pain relief and about the fact that no one and nothing can relieve my pain, not even morphine.

It torments me to think about one specific day, an afternoon at the stables, when you'd invited me to watch your riding lesson. We'd just arrived and you were searching for Tampa, your lopsided horse, the one with the wild streak, who was bowlegged, who no one wanted, and who you had looked after and put back on track. You were the only one who gave him food and brushed his tail, you'd managed to get him to jump over one-meter-high obstacles and you wanted to prepare him for a competition. But Tampa wasn't there—and all the stalls were full. They'd released him in the field toward the hills and it had rained, and now he was nowhere to be found.

I was there with you while you cried, the brush for his mane in your hand, his saddle hanging on the hook. The horse wasn't yours. You couldn't pay to keep him in a stall. He was just a hobby horse, and you'd told me: Tampa isn't used to being in the field and they didn't shoe him properly, he'll hurt himself, he'll cripple himself. And I didn't have any solutions or answers, I wasn't able to console you. I'd just stood there watching you cry and observing your desperation—I didn't lift a finger to let you know I understood you'd been wronged and that I would resolve it, avenge it. That I would find the money for ten, twenty horses, and I would build stables that were yours and yours alone, where you could give all the animals names and teach them to be elegant and fast. Instead I'd simply said: Horses are used to being in the fields, I don't think he'll get hurt out in the open air. And you had withdrawn, offended by my incomprehension. It wasn't about that horse, it wasn't about the competition, and it wasn't about not having enough money, it was that no one seemed to care about hurting you.

You'd walked right past me, grabbed your riding cap, and went out to the field. You climbed on another horse that belonged to an Englishwoman who didn't feel like riding it every day, and with that horse you'd gone around and around—at a walk, at a trot, at a canter—and I felt like I could see a curse on your face the entire time. I stood off to the side, watching you stir up dust. I'd started coughing and then moved over to the shade, among the flies and the weeds.

The next day, we found out that Tampa had in fact crippled himself and they'd soon be putting him down.

I didn't ask if I could join you to say goodbye—you hadn't expressed any desire for me to be there. You'd gone alone to the euthanization, and your face was dark for days afterward. To try to lift your spirits, Agata invited you to the stables where she often went, to choose a new horse. There were some young ones who needed to be trained, and you'd said: It's not the same.

And that's what torments me, because no, it's not the same.

It's not the same without Tampa. It's not the same without you.

This letter sucks—it's worse than my compositions for school. You won't receive it and I won't send it. It might as well not exist.

But you asked me to write it, so here it is, this pointless letter.
I miss you and I've been a terrible, terrible, terrible friend.

Yours,
Gaia

During the fish festival, the lakefront is filled with balloons, mothers in high heels, and fried pike heads. The beach was closed off in anticipation of the fireworks that start at midnight. In the past, I would watch them from the sand, but that's been prohibited ever since the time some debris landed on a lady and her straw hat caught fire. The little kids got scared, and we laughed, happy to witness a bit of danger.

People stroll back and forth from the Chalet restaurant to behind the Soldati. People crowd together, suck on candies and swallow them, stop at the bars to buy pizzette, and take photos of themselves leaning on the railings. Kids wink at one another to say hello, and the people you haven't seen all winter come back into your life. If there's any event that can't be missed, it's this one.

On a wooden stage, amateur performances take place one after the other: dance recitals, improvisational singers, girls in sequins and hair spray, and a comedian cracking greasy smiles. The seats in the first row are almost always empty, and some of the performers are practically invisible next to the noisy promenade.

My favorite place to sit and watch the fireworks is from the flat roof of a stranger's house, which I can get to by climbing over the railings of the small park right below town hall. It has a clear view of the lake, without any tall antennae or bulky trees, perfect for

watching the fireworks explode: the artificial hearts, the weeping wil-
lows, the yellow stars, the big booms that make kids cover their ears,
the fountains of light rising up in the night, the dense smoke, the
debris of burnt paper left on the water's surface. People come from
the towns all around the lake and even from Rome to see how well
we light up the sky.

The streets are closed off and there are long lines of parked cars.
People proceed single file along the asphalt banks, little children in
their arms, strollers under their armpits, skirts held up with two fingers to avoid the grass and dust. Some women put on special makeup
for the fish festival, tease their hair, straighten their bangs, wear lace-
up sandals, and buy T-shirts with deep V-necks for the occasion.
They stuff their bras and keep their sunglasses on top of their heads
even when there's no sun.

I reach the pier on my bike, racing downhill from the Cross.
Like a missile, I swoop down on all the families and create space
for myself to land, then I turn behind a restaurant and lock up my
bike. I have the ravenous eyes of a wolf. I see them all dressed up
for their celebration and feel like there's no respect, no sympathy.
They're dressed colorfully and wearing flowers. No one is here for
my mourning.

I didn't have to make anything up—my clothes are almost all
black. The only thing that isn't black is my hair. Its color bothers me
in the mirror. How dare it stay red, carnal, thriving, while everything
else in my body is drying up? Who said it could keep living?

I walk through the alleyways, avoiding the Piazza del Molo where
huddles of teenagers remind me that my youth has passed me by, the
sluggish and dormant years, the best years, swallowed up by life like
a season come to its end.

I walk with my head down, eyes fixed on the cobblestones, and my small shoulder bag banging against my hip. People laugh, but what are they laughing at? Why are they laughing? Two people I know walk by and their eyes widen. They see my hard face and don't dare say hello. I gather from their expressions that they already know everything, and I hate them for their knowledge. This town can't keep a secret, not even when it comes to death, when it comes to pain.

I want to head up the stone stairs to the small park, climb over the railing, and wait by myself for midnight to come. It's almost here. That rooftop is my eternal return, my point of contact with the past, my circular time—the view is always the same. The sounds, too. When the fireworks go off, I'll have the illusion of eternity, where everything condenses and nothing elapses, and Iris and I will still be sitting there together with our legs crossed and the lights in our eyes.

A girl stops me. She's dressed as a majorette. Her short dress hugs her hips and she has big, long arms. I recognize her—she's the younger sister of a girl who went to high school with Iris. She has a small, pronounced chin and feline eyes. She observes me and seems penitent, ready to lift her knees and thighs to march, do pirouettes. She mumbles: I heard, I'm so sorry, she was such a beautiful girl . . .

Her condolences feel like a bullet to the back of my head. I awaken from my reveries and snap back to reality, and the reality is that people look at me with pity and stop me to share their ritual words because yes—she was a beautiful girl and they put her riding boots on her and then they burned her.

So I push her—that disgraceful, puny little body in front of me. It breathes, it moves—how dare she exist? I yell back that no one died and we don't need her horrible sympathy. I claw my way toward her

and attack. Her friends jump between us. Other people stop and try
to pull me away, and I continue to defend Iris and myself from their
disease, from their duplicity. Here you all are, dressed up for the evening, polished and painted, ready to make your toasts.

I feel the smooth fabric of her dress between my fingers and I
want to yank it off and tear it to pieces: the street parade with the
band, the stalls selling earthenware, the candied nuts, the princess-
shaped balloons, the greasy paper cones dripping oil, the steam rising
toward the houses . . . I try to free myself but someone is holding me
tightly by the shoulders and saying I have to stay calm. He says *calm*
once more and holds me back.

I recognize the voice and yell out: Cristia', do something!

He holds me as the girl is rescued from my nails and my claws,
my monstrous face. People crowd around us. She's frightened and
crying, and I ask Cristiano again to do something because he has
to be capable of resolving this. He always arrives at exactly the
right moment, brings matches and gasoline, knows how to lead me
unharmed through the dark, silences whoever is trying to accuse me,
protects me from betrayals, has a gun ready to fire. We have to strike
something or someone, take revenge for the wrong I've suffered.

What do you think you're looking at? Cristiano, holding the lump
of flesh that I am in his arms—sweaty and pale and limp—drives
people away.

I feel like there has to be a reason Iris died. Maybe it's the pre-
servatives, maybe the polyphosphates, maybe the greenhouse gases,
maybe the pesticides, maybe the burnt plastic, maybe the radiation
from the antennae, maybe it's Radio Vaticana, maybe it's the arsenic in the water, maybe it's the fiber cement in the roofs of the
houses, maybe the waves emitted by cell phones and Wi-Fi, maybe

the hormones in meat, maybe the active smoking and secondhand smoke, maybe the synthetic feed given to chickens and cows, maybe the tar at the mouths of rivers, maybe the smog from the cars, maybe it's the sewage, maybe the medicines and the medical waste, maybe the silicone in body lotions, maybe the additives and the paints— maybe. We have to find the culprits, each and every one of her murderers. We have to.

Cristiano holds my forehead and leads me over to the fountain. He keeps saying to all the people coming up to us that we don't need any help, and he splashes water on my face.

There's nothing I can do, he tells me. My dress is wet, my bag is underwater, and my Motorola has slipped to the ground, it's floating in a puddle.

In the meantime, three shots go off, announcing the start of the fireworks, and they reverberate throughout the basin of our town. You can hear them from the countryside, the borgo antico, the Collegiata church, the fish market, the fried-fish stalls, maybe as far away as Pizzo Bend. One, two, three—and the show begins.

⁓

At the end of the sixties, the Germans discovered the old part of our town, the borgo antico, the part that's high up and perched near the tower and gardens that were once an outpost of the Odescalchi Castle, offering a lookout over the lake.

There the narrow cobblestone streets lead all the way up to the Collegiata, the church for important weddings, with the priest who loudly reprimands witnesses for their revealing dresses. Substantial offerings are required to get married there because if you don't pay, the priest takes away the music and the bride is forced to enter in silence, accompanied only by the photographer's clicks and the children's giggles.

The borgo antico, where there are still a few shops and bars with plastic chairs occupied by old people and town hall employees. The borgo, which is accessed through a huge wooden door that's almost always wide open. There are three restaurants, the studio of a glass-jewelry designer, and a tabaccheria. The tattoo parlors and windsurf shops have come and gone, but the shoemakers and the fountain with the open-mouthed eels have lasted.

The Germans delighted in those ramshackle little houses with bedrooms on the lower floors and kitchens right at the entrances, balconies overlooking the lake and small stone columns, the ancient smell of the walls.

They bought houses and stores, opened businesses, then quickly closed them—this town doesn't like new things. It's more interested in conserving and maintaining, like the viscous liquid of a preservative, sealing casks and barrels.

The Germans looked for work in the city, went down to the little beaches below the borgo antico and stretched out naked in the sun, ate panini with herring, and bought themselves straw hats. The people in town hated them. They detested them like metastasis, like they were illnesses, like something that needed to be eradicated.

The Germans thought the lake was beautiful. They saw how it attracted the sun and all the colors, how it melded with the sky, so they brought two white swans from their country to make the lake more sophisticated.

The two swans were superb animals with regal plumage, tame and innocuous at first glance. But the townspeople couldn't bear the indignity of watching foreigners change the fauna of their lake, when everything was meant to stay as it was, like a painting hung on the wall.

The fishermen started saying the swans were toxic, they carried diseases, they ate all the fish, they killed the other birds. The swans were filthy and murderous.

One day, instead of going fishing, two fishermen with rowboats and small nets caught the swans and strangled them. They cooked them, and the smoke from their flesh rose from the trees below the borgo antico, along that strip of land where no one could walk because the path ends much earlier.

The Germans mourned their children with the broad wings and pointed beaks, but they didn't lose heart. To introduce new things, you need to be stubborn. Bringing about change calls for perseverance, a dose of mania.

Other swans arrived and were again roasted, then more and more followed, and the townspeople watched them splash around and procreate, and without even realizing it they began to like those large, imperial animals who managed to keep the ducks and their ducklings in line.

And so the swans stayed, and they moved from one shore to the next. There's a black one on the Bracciano coastline, below the castle. It's the only one that never approaches people. These days, over forty years later, children search for swans along the shore, eager to feed them stale bread and stroke their feathers. But swans, of course, aren't pond birds. They aren't rule followers and they're easily angered. When you see one, you have to know how far away to stay.

One of the first things I learned when I arrived was this: You can approach ducks without worry, but not swans. Swans peck at the backs of nutrias and chase them into the water, flapping their wings. Swans don't differentiate between young girls and adult women—if they dislike you, they will hurt you. I was a swan. They brought me here from elsewhere, and I had to find my place out of necessity. I harassed, kicked, and fought even those who approached me with their chunk of hard bread, their offering of love.

I look at them now, on the lakefront, diving under the water in search of food. Only the tips of their tails stay afloat; their heads disappear. When they come back up, they look at me as if to say the algae on the bottom isn't as good as it used to be—it might even be time to migrate.

Home is where things fall to the floor.

We've already broken three plates, two glasses, and one of the cupboard's glass panes. The milk carton fell and formed a pale puddle in the center of the kitchen.

Antonia arranged the boxes they gave her at the supermarket in a row along the hallway. As usual, nothing is packed randomly. Everything is securely stacked, perfectly positioned. Each box is closed tightly with tape, and we write what each of them contains in marker: toothbrushes go with toothbrushes, curtains with curtains. Books ended up in the black bag my mother gave me, without her realizing it, along with the waste and refuse.

She's the captain of our ship, guiding us, staying the course, giving orders, and imparting discipline—even when a storm appears on the horizon, when something slips through the cracks. It's gone now, she says. Broken objects will be abandoned; we'll only save what is whole and indispensable. For the first time, we, too, throw things out. We don't rebuild, we don't redecorate, we don't glue back together, we don't repaint.

The twins wrap up our television set with the same care one would show a marble statuette, and my father watches them, apprehensive. He fears a crack, some kind of slippage, the end of his reign.

I stuffed my clothes into two large bags, and in a corner I piled all the things my body rejects: the skintight skirts, low-rise jeans, pants with holes in the butt, bras missing a strap—all the scraps I'd held on to, obsessed by the thought that sooner or later they'd have a second chance. But now they appear to me as what they really are: rags, tights worn over and over again to the point of exhaustion, T-shirts with armpit stains that not even Antonia's hands can wash out, the black bathing suit from that one brilliant summer that's now faded and stained, yellowed underwear, hems eaten away from rubbing against asphalt, the Superman T-shirt that smells like ash.

I finally threw out the tennis racket, after inhaling its scent one last time and running my fingers along it, strumming it like a lyre and kissing it. I said farewell to the racket and farewell to Ears. I loved and hated you both until today.

I should have a house of my own, children of my own, a marriage of my own, a job of my own, and instead I'm gathering up what's left of a child's bedroom. I detach the string from the walls that had been left hanging there long after the sheets dividing my half of the room from Mariano's had been taken down. I gather up a pair of my brother's underwear and his basketball, the top of one of his pajama sets with elephants on it, his posters of singers, the Che Guevara flag, the sheets that have been left waiting for him under his comforter for years, his high school notebooks containing his rough, exaggerated handwriting.

We're leaving marks on the walls, mildew in the corners, nails sticking out that no longer hold anything on them, holes where the shelves used to be, stained tiles, grout lines with traces of blood, dust, hair, dead skin, nail clippings.

That's staying here, my mother orders, pointing at the pink bear. Stuffed animals are for children. You don't need it. Then she walks out of the room.

She doesn't even wait for my response. It's been like this for a long time. Whatever she says goes. Dialogue isn't permitted, sharing anything is impossible. When I told her Iris was dead, she replied: To lose a child is the greatest heartache, then she stood up and went off to trim the green beans, and that's how our commemoration ended, our outpouring of grief.

Antonia has grown more compact and more wiry. She's lost her physical stamina and much of her spirit. She faces everything with a certain bitterness. She does not tolerate disorder or resistance.

For months, I've heard her moving around the house at night, making agitated phone calls, yelling, throwing her hands up in the air, striking tables and other hard surfaces.

Signora Mirella Mancini, née Boretti, is renting out the apartment in Rome, and the tenants, who don't even have leases, aren't paying their rent. They're not paying the bills. Both the building manager and the doorwoman informed my mother, asking her for the money that's owed them. She called Signora Mirella, but didn't get a response, so she kept calling, only to be ignored. When she finally got through, the signora said she was willing to fight. If

292 · GIULIA CAMINITO

my mother didn't stop bothering her, she would get her custody of Corso Trieste taken away, because she could do that, she had contacts, she knew people, while Antonia, on the other hand, was all alone—with her rotten family, no job contract, and everyone dependent on her.

My mother didn't eat or sleep that day. When I got up in the middle of the night to go to the bathroom, I found her sitting on the couch, staring at the blank TV screen, reflected in the darkness.

The next morning, she gathered us all in the kitchen to tell us she'd spoken to the Festas' gardener, Giacomo, a trustworthy man. He'd come pick us up in a week. We had to work quickly and empty out the apartment.

That woman thinks I'll give up. She thinks she's tricked me, but I'll occupy that house. I want to see someone try to take me away. Her face began to contort.

She divided the tasks among us and marked the days on the calendar—seven—before our departure.

The doorwoman and building manager were notified. We were coming back. Signora Mirella got the notice, too. My mother had written her a long message full of bad grammar, but the threats were clear—she had one week to get the boarders out of our house, or else my mother would do it herself, with her own two hands.

The twins didn't complain. They were dutiful in gathering their things, tall now and with large hands, almost men already with hair on their chins and their own desires. Squeezed into clothes from two winters prior, they were ready to sort through things and pack up, and in their secret language of glances and furtive gestures, they halfheartedly tell each other that they will survive this.

I don't have time to observe our empty house in all its nakedness—its cracks and its memories, its skin, the crooks of its elbows, its belly button. I'm dragged outside by my mother's wrath, which, like a current, carries all the sticks, stones, and snakes toward the delta. This river never slows.

I'm a young and yet somehow already old woman. I've lost the right to oppose our family's movements, though I never really had it. It's as if I missed my stop and am now forced to stay on until the end of the line. No one thought to ask me for my opinion or to include me in the most important decisions. Antonia is the same mother from my childhood, the one who single-handedly holds up the walls when they threaten to collapse and carries us out of the burning house on her back.

I close the door to my room and behind it I find the orange poster from my eighteenth birthday. There are photos of Iris, photos of Agata, photos of me, and there's Babol's snout, worn down by the years and by its own futility, a trophy that weighs the same as a medal one might win at a cross-country race. From a distance, that moment of victory and power is nothing but dust.

On Monday, the closets are emptied; Tuesday, the bathroom; Wednesday, the kitchen cabinets; Thursday is for the rugs and textiles; Friday, we throw out the trash bags; Saturday, we clean the floors and bathroom fixtures. By Sunday, we're ready to leave.

The piazzale with the carnival and the swing ride, the streets, the roads, the stores, the railroad crossings—we leave everything behind, and the distance from who we once were grows. The vans carrying everything we own set out for a house we may no longer be able to have and leave behind a house we've just cleared out.

294 · GIULIA CAMINITO

Once we're in Rome, Antonia has the vans double-park next to the apartment building on Corso Trieste and she gets out, her muscles tense, her red hair in a high ponytail, her down jacket zipped up to her chin, and her face smooth and poisonous. She has them open the gates to let us in—the gates stolen from the Fascists. They're reminders that this building has a history.

Roberta died four years ago in her sleep—she just stopped breathing. I look over at her corner of sun, where today there is only shadow. I see the fish fountain emptied of water and filled with succulents, the courtyard and the roses—yellow, red, and salmon colored. Many of the residents have changed. The building has filled up with B&Bs and vacation rentals, students who share rooms, and families with few children. There was never any danger of the property value depreciating. Rome's housing market always yields gains, and now that there are fewer jobs, renting out apartments has become a job in itself.

Antonia carries a toolbox up the stairs to the landing. Everything looks foreign; everything seems to have been waiting for our return.

Our last name is no longer on the doorbell. Instead, there's a white nameplate and a red, felted doormat. My mother moves it aside brusquely with her foot. The lock has been changed and the door bolted shut.

This house is ours! she shouts into the stairwell, for the neighbors who've stuck their heads out, the curious, the fearful. We'll be out here until we can get inside.

I feel incompetent and don't know how to help. I'm ashamed of our shortcomings. Here is yet another struggle that takes us back to the days of our first home in the basement, back to when it wasn't written down anywhere that we were deserving of shelter.

Signora Mirella had two wooden planks nailed across the door, like a building declared uninhabitable, like some dilapidated farmhouse or a basement filled with needles and condoms. The twins pull out their tools and start tinkering, guided by Antonia, and their thin, adolescent wrists hold up the hammers and pliers as best they can.

My mother doesn't ask me to do anything. She lets me be a mere spectator of their efforts. The planks won't move, the nails won't budge. They seem to rage against destiny and the orbits of the planets.

Antonia's hands tremble, but she doesn't stop. She says she'll ram into the door with her shoulder over and over until it breaks open, she'll come back with dynamite if she needs to. She's been left behind for her entire life, but no longer. It's going to take all the saints in heaven to stop her. She attacks the nails and the wall, strikes the plaster and the lime, attempts to find the hinges and pounds the jambs and planks with loud blows.

I'm thinking about the fish: Were they released into the sewers? Maybe now they're swimming under the manholes, searching for the still very distant sea. Maybe they've mutated and each have three eyes and five fins. They've been contaminated by our fabric softeners, antilimescale dishwasher tablets, bathroom sanitizers, and chamomile, white musk, and shea butter shampoos.

Then we hear some people coming up the stairs, and one of them yells out: Ma'!

My mother stops. Her knuckles are red, her forehead wet, and her face looks bewildered when she sees her son arrive.

Move over, Ma'. We'll take care of it.

Mariano joins us on the landing. He's brought three friends who are all tall and large and dark like him. They're carrying metal pipes, crowbars, and have scarves pulled up over their faces. We step back and let them through. At the first strike Mariano gives to the door, my mother shudders in silence, pressed up against the elevator.

The nails and planks jump. The concrete jumps, too, and Mariano uses a crowbar to strip the hinges, applying pressure with his hands and legs. Meanwhile, his friends force the door, hitting it with everything they've got until my brother can tell that it's finally giving in. He rams into it with his shoulder, one two three five times—his body slamming into the door—until it cracks and a hole opens up. Through it, you can see the house.

My brother's nose is smeared with white dust. Plaster from the wall covers his fingers and clothes, and blood is dripping from one hand. His jacket sleeve is torn, but he doesn't give up. Again and again, he kicks the lock until a passage is made. He crosses the threshold, plunging into our past.

His friends follow him in, my mother goes in, the twins go in, and they are all swallowed up by that toothless mouth. I go in last. Signora Mirella had battered the bottom of the bathtub and the built-in kitchen, sliced the sofa upholstery open with scissors, and taken things that weren't hers—things my mother had left in the house as part of their fair exchange. She'd had the electrical wiring cut and detached the curtain rods from above the windows. Our house looks like a construction site, a crime scene.

Mariano walks around to evaluate the damage. He's already entered the second phase, the triage stage. He's thinking about how to help the house heal from its wounds, its scratches, from the violence. He says they'll take care of the door and the tub first, then figure out how to fix things in the kitchen, and they'll sew the sofa back together. In the meantime, we should carry our furniture and the rest of our things upstairs, then they'll patrol outside the building, in front of our door—no one else will be allowed to enter. My mother nods, she looks at him with eyes full of gratitude. There's no one who could have saved us if not my brother, because he's just like her. Here I was under the impression that my resemblance to my mother—hair, freckles, nose—was a sign of our closeness. Instead, it's right in front of me, once again: our utter inconsistency.

Mariano orders me: Don't just stand there with that look on your face, help Mamma. He says this to me as though I were some worker at his construction site, a delivery boy running behind schedule, or a wife who can't seem to get pregnant.

Then he races down the stairs and shouts that he's going to get his father.

I observe the disaster as if it were snow that had simply fallen on us—the air is cold, the view blinding. My brother is a mountain and I am a grasshopper. For a moment, I wish he would hug me, but he doesn't and I don't ask him to.

Mariano reemerges from the smashed-in door, carrying Massimo in his arms. He had to leave his chair outside the door. He arranges my father's legs one at a time, his little, broken legs, and says: It's okay, Papà.

My father is crying. My father has seen our damaged house.

Mariano keeps his bloody hand steady on Massimo's shoulder and tells him it's not over.

I'm motionless and I meet the eyes of the girl I once was. I look at myself in the cracked mirror above the bathroom sink and whisper: There's no home for the heartless.

The lake is dry. They said so on television. During the summer, Rome sucked up water from the lake for its own supply, so the beaches have gotten longer, stones have emerged, pilings have surfaced, the rocks look like islands, and to be able to go underwater, you have to walk and walk, far from the beach and the shouting, far from any possibility of being saved.

People in town think the lake will disappear and that Rome will take away more water each summer until it turns into a puddle, a foul-smelling basin resembling marshland, and only then will we really see what's in the middle—whether the submerged city with its walls, courtyards, and windows will return to the world.

The Corso Trieste house was painted and repaired. Like a broken doll, they fixed her arms and legs, brushed her tangled hair, and put her little dress and apron back on. The house is once again habitable. We sleep in our beds, the television is back in its proper place against the wall, the boxes have been emptied, the sofas repaired with colorful patches, the trinkets have reappeared, as well as my mother's inventions—the doors with the decoupage, the cacti in yogurt containers.

Mariano paces back and forth between the sofa and the front doorway, always on the lookout, always on guard. He spends the evenings sitting at the table with my mother; they plan and scheme. They know exactly what needs to be done.

She has to start working, I heard them say. They were talking about me.

We need money we don't have to properly care for our home, so one day my mother handed me a vacuum and a bucket with rags, detergent, and a pair of gloves inside, and she told me: Go to the signora on the sixth floor. It's time to clean her house.

So I went up to her apartment, with its ethnic armchairs, floor-to-ceiling bookshelves, framed photographs, Capodimonte porcelain, ivory candelabras, vinyl records, dusty ladders, collection of stones from around the world, old magazines in the bathroom, wrought-iron bed frames, wicker baskets, portrait of a woman with one exposed breast, chandeliers that look like sculptures, dried flowers perfuming the rooms, shoeboxes all lined up, document holders full of old bills, Murano glassware, teacups from a museum in Canada, basil plant on the balcony, and figurine of a frog sitting on a tree trunk.

My mother told me to clean as if it were my house, so I cleaned angrily and got carried away with the stains in the shower (wide, yellow, distressing), all the dust in the crevices, and the hair on the floor next to the bedside tables.

Now I'm alone in our house. Mariano brought my father outside to wander around the neighborhood; he had him put on a sweater so he doesn't get cold and placed a cap with a brim on his head. My father was agitated but happy—happy that his son was with him and taking care of everything, from excursions like these to the electricity, from broken doors to gas pipes. This is what sons do: they put the world and the future in order.

From far, far away, I hear the echo of my dives, of my jumps into the water. My bicycle stayed in Anguillara, as did my bear Babol, Cristiano, and the urn with Iris inside—with her spleen and her kneecaps and her irises—and now I feel like a crater has opened in the center of my chest where there had once been a volcano. Who can say? Over centuries it will rain, and in the end, someone will call it a lake, though it was once just a hole, the ghost of something that has faded away.

If I had a car, I'd travel across the city to then leave it behind and return to the sounds of the Monday market, to red paddleboats moving slowly, to shrimp-and-salmon pizzas, to beach umbrellas planted in the sand with the help of shovels and feet, to inflatable toys hanging outside of a newsstand, making little girls anxious. But I'm stuck here, and here is where I've arrived.

I stand up and move around creakily. I'm rusty. I've been exposed too long to the winds and the rains. I'm guided by thoughts that write novels, that distort realities.

I remember when I'd just arrived, when everything felt big and grand to me, when these spacious rooms felt like whole houses, and when poorly lit basements were the landscapes of my childhood. I remember the twins running around on their short, chubby legs, their diapers swishing, and how they clung to Antonia's thighs. I remember me, Mariano, and Antonia, united in the courtyard with our underwear and shame exposed. Like tortoises, we fought against small injustices, against those who didn't want us there. I remember the me who wanted roses from other people's gardens so I could chop them up and torture them, make slime out of them, and reproduce expensive essences. I remember my mother telling me what was bad and what was good, and she believed what she was saying—that it's possible to split the world in two.

I walk into the bathroom. The tub has been replaced. It's white and shiny like the most pristine teeth. I turn the faucets on all the way. I can already smell the algae and whitefish and swans.

Then I move on to the sink and the bidet. The water comes out in a torrent. It's impossible not to hear it flowing. I plug the drains and the water starts to pool, rising a few centimeters at a time.

When the lake is completely drained, we'll debunk the legends, the lies, the stories. We'll discover artifacts, place antiquities in display cases, watch fish struggle in the open air, and understand the color of the earth that we never get to see. We'll recover all the lost fishing poles, sunken boats, deflated life jackets, drowned cadavers, crashed helicopter propellers, and we'll finally stop thinking about it all. We'll stop fishing and pulling up nets, stop hiding nativity scenes and rifles underwater.

It's time to move on to the kitchen that my brother patched up with lime and tiles. I heard him, day and night, messing around with the putty knife in a bucket. I turn on that faucet, too, and plug the drain. I leave the doors to all the rooms wide open, letting in air, letting in water, letting myself in, too.

I sit down in the middle of the living room and wonder how much time it will take—whether two, three, seven hours will be enough, whether I will, at a certain point, be able to feel the water reach my ankles, or at least the tips of my toes—the stolen lake water, the bitter and perfect lake water, the water that will form troublesome puddles, that will gush and dampen, that will create stains on the ceilings below, slip into the cracks and then leak and soak sofas and bedside tables, bottles of oil, books and catalogs, magazines, trash bags, dust jackets, curtains. The water will bother the bystanders. It will reach the foundation. It will become a plague. The water will invade the street and the neighborhood, the cars will be submerged and people will have to build themselves rafts and shelters, leave their belongings behind and their properties unattended. Those who can't stay afloat will be carried away.

I close my eyes and begin to count.

Lake Is a Magical Word

You're coming from the main road and you cross the fields of yellow grass. You pass a few used-car dealerships, a gas station, and on the left, you catch a glimpse of a junkyard selling wrought-iron rocking chairs and bedside tables with brass knobs.

You go past the brush and rocks, and you stop in the middle of the road because you hear the signal: the railroad crossing is closing. You line up behind other cars with open windows. Some turn off their motors. Trains in the countryside take turns; there is no double track like in the city. Here, they have to give each other the right of way, and the railroad crossing can stay closed for up to ten minutes, but there's no way around it. Wherever you're going, even on the side streets, you'll find the crossing gate down.

The railway is the only way out for those who don't have cars, it's the aorta that pumps blood, the horizon, the threshold of adventure. On a train you first arrived, and on a train you kept leaving.

When the barrier goes back up, you drive slowly over the tracks. If you turn your head to the right, you can see the train station's shelters. You took that train for years—you know every car, every spray-painted graffiti, all the tags written with Uni Posca markers. You remember the crowded cars, the people packed in tight. You remember when a pregnant woman fainted in the crowd, and when they raped a girl at La Storta. You remember when you would hold the doors open so your friends could get on, when you didn't have a ticket and would run to the end of the train and hide in the bathrooms, when you met a boy older than you with alcohol on his breath, carrying cucumbers in a glass jar and bread for the swans in his bag.

The main road continues, lined with stores. There's the fruit-and-vegetable stand that also sells snails, the huge furniture factory that offers expensive kitchens and cutting-edge lamps, the supermarkets and the fish markets—it's what they call the station neighborhood, the urban part of town, where there are houses, basement gyms, and a bar that makes nachos and tortillas at night. Right along the main road are the commercial businesses. Farther in, there are houses with two floors, at most, and slides in the yards.

You don't want to stop. You pass the pharmacy and the office of your family doctor. You slow down at the crosswalk and let a woman cross with a young boy. He stares at you as if you were a vampire.

A moment later, you're in the Residenza Claudia neighborhood. They call it that because of the Claudia Spring, with its natural mineral water.

On the left, a piazzale opens up and that's where the public housing is—nondescript multistory buildings—and there on the third
floor is your house, though it can't really be called yours anymore.
There's the window of your room, the tree from which Bear broke a
branch, the railing where you'd lock up your bicycle, the clearing for
the carnival rides around Easter, the shooting gallery, the shots going
off, the cans falling, you and Mariano climbing the stairs, one holding
the head and the other holding the paws of an enormous pink bear.

Every storefront reminds you of an afternoon. Their functions
have all changed over the years, from dentistry to orthopedics, from
selling footwear to fresh flowers, from frozen foods to household
items, from everything for one euro to handmade ceramics, from
dog grooming to cell phone service. You feel a need to stay loyal to
those that have been around the longest.

You've crossed this intersection in all directions over the years. It's
where the one and only glorious traffic light in all of town is. Waiting
for it to turn green was part of your adolescence. If you turned right,
you could head down the street where the hotel pool is and go back
in there, in a bathing suit and robe, stand still in the locker room, with
your hairbrush, your bottle of eucalyptus shampoo, and see Carlotta
again, hear her say: Here I am.

Farther that way, driving around the Residenza Claudia neighborhood, you could also go see the piazzetta and the old abandoned
house, which they've now restored. A family lives there: they have
three children, a dog, two canaries. Continuing on, you'd arrive in
front of Andrea's house, where the gate is black from smoke, and on
the street corners there are still signs of the fire. Soon he'll be getting
married. They've already printed the invitations. His future wife is a
dentist and she's very blonde.

But you don't want to turn, so you wait for the green. If you're lucky, it won't take long to get through the intersection and then on the right you'll see a big farmhouse, so different from the rest of the buildings it seems alien—an old country house along the road of a place that wants to become a city, it's a reminder of a former world.

This is where the bad thoughts begin for you. You see the little street that climbs up from the main road. Halfway up that hill there was and perhaps always will be Iris's house. You traveled that street on foot, by bike, by car, with the stereo on, with the windows up, at night, arguing, saying unfair things, loving, and you feel like you can still see the imprint of the bag full of lemons in front of the gate.

So don't turn there. Stay on the main road and keep going because the main road will always arrive at the lake, and that is where you need to go.

Never mind the cemetery on your right. Don't think about the graves, don't think about the photo they chose for Carlotta—a cut-out. In the original one, you were there next to her and you couldn't bring yourself to smile. You're getting closer and closer, you can see the first buildings of the historical center, you can see the sign for the pastry shop where you used to stop for late-night croissants and sandwiches.

You've almost arrived at the Cross, the most famous intersection in town, where people who come from the countryside sometimes park with their horses just to show everyone they can leave them tied to a pole while they go for coffee. Even Cristiano has done it. He took someone's horse just for the sake of riding it into town. Cristiano, who renovated his farm and now has quite a few goats, cows, and calves, and makes a good aged cheese, one they use in restaurants.

If you go left from the Cross, you find two streets named after saints, San Francesco and Santo Stefano. The first is the one that leads to the middle and elementary schools. It's the street many take to go to mass, and in summer, there's also an open-air cinema that way. The other leads to the houses of the wealthy—the biggest ones, built high up, looking down on the lake and the historical center—new villas with large gardens, tall trees, automatic gates. You've never had a gate of your own and you envy them—the people who have remote controls, who only need to go *click* to enter.

If you turn right at the Cross, you head toward Trevignano and basically end up at the lake. You can drive alongside it, keep going where the houses thin out, where there are bamboo canes and inlets. It's a calm area that makes you think of Cristiano's moped and the headlights turned off—the dark comes and those who survive are the ones who know the bends in the road and the stop signs by heart, who dodge the ditches, who brake in time.

Deciding to go straight instead, you've arrived.

You can enter the borgo antico, walk down the alleyways, climb up to the Collegiata church, ask someone to marry you, put on a white strapless dress, or you can head downhill to the lake.

Your choice—this is where we leave you. We'll pull over, tell you to get out, and you'll go on foot.

Now you seem to be in a hurry: Run by the jewelry shop where you and Iris wanted to get your ears pierced together, pass the pizzeria with the eighties decor and the smelly waiter, don't think about all those laps you've done back and forth along the promenade on mopeds, in cars, on foot, your eyes on everyone, and everyone's eyes on you. Keep running, all the way to the pier, then take off your clothes—the striped T-shirt, the black jeans, the sneakers worn down at the toes. Climb over the railing, launch yourself onto one of the pilings. Be careful. It's slippery.

Now look behind you. There's someone waiting for you. Offer her your hand and keep your promise.

Tell her not to lean out too far. First she has to find her balance and gain control of her own weight. Beneath you is the water of January, of April, of August—it's the water you used to stare at, searching for Christ's reflection. It's proof that you drove all this way just to jump. Close your eyes and tell her to do the same, then shout: Lake is a magical word!

Only after shouting do you and Iris find the courage to jump.

Author's Note

This novel was written to tell the story of three women through three characters inspired by them. The first is Antonella, who shared her family's story with me—about their fight for housing, a house exchange, and how she eventually managed, after years of struggles, to reclaim their lost home. I took some creative license with her story—like using Anguillara Sabazia, for instance. I don't believe the municipality of Rome has any public housing there.

The second woman is Ilaria, who was my best friend for ten years. She was sarcastic and stubborn, knew how to make pastry cream and ride horses in the woods, loved bunnies and *Anna Karenina*. She died in 2015.

The third woman is me. I never hit a boy with a racket, never tried to drown Elena in the lake, never won a pink bear at a carnival, and

I certainly don't know how to shoot—I'm even afraid when I'm alone at night. This is not a biography, an autobiography, or a work of autofiction—this is a story that swallowed up many fragments of many lives and tried to weave a narrative out of them. It's the story of the years of my youth, of sorrows I only skirted around, as well as those I experienced firsthand.

I want to thank Anguillara Sabazia, which serves as the backdrop for this novel, and all those who live there. I want to thank Lake Bracciano, the lost city of Sabazia, the sunsets in Vicarello, the Air Force Museum, the Vigna di Valle sailing clubs, the Trevignano promenade, the Gabbiano bar, the PepeNero open-air discoteca, the Pioppo public beach, Pizzo Bend, the shuttle bus that connects the lakefront to the train station, the regional trains on the Viterbo–Roma Tiburtina route, the Monday market, and the shops that are always closed on Thursdays. I want to thank Pedro Cano and the borgo antico, the Collegiata and San Biagio churches, Angela Zucconi and the library dedicated to her, the Movida summer parties in Bracciano, the Orsini-Odescalchi Castle, the eels I've never seen and the swans I used to always see, the downhill dirt road that leads to Martignano, the Due Laghi stables, and all the other spots around the lake that I've loved. I want to thank the Sagra del Pesce fish festival and the fried fish, the fireworks and the roofs we watched them from, the dance recitals held on lopsided stages, all the singers who performed and were listened to by very few people.

I want to thank those who betrayed me, those who mocked me, those who hated me, and those who understood me, who hugged me. I want to thank my friends who are alive and who cherish these memories along with me. I want to thank those who worked behind the scenes on this book, those who were extras without wanting to be, those whose implicit or explicit quotations I stole, and those who might get upset reading this. I want to thank Laura Fidaleo, because her words are the magical ones I started with.

Lastly, I want to share several truths:

In 2012, Federica Mangiapelo was a victim of femicide, drowned by her boyfriend in the waters of Lake Bracciano on the night of Halloween. She was sixteen years old.

In 2017, Pope Francis disconnected most of the Radio Vaticana antennae after they were accused of having caused an increase in malignant tumors and leukemia cases in the children of the surrounding area.

Also in 2017, in Kraków, the UNESCO committee approved the inclusion of the Oriolo Romano beech forest in the World Heritage List, though the area remains plagued by poaching.

In 2019, the Roman industrial company ACEA was banned from extracting water from Lake Bracciano. Still today, the Anguillara Sabazia aqueducts are periodically declared dangerous because they contain levels of arsenic exceeding permissible limits. Over the years, valuable archaeological findings have emerged from the lake, including tangible proof of submerged villas and houses.

And, in any case, I have never seen that nativity scene in the water under the pier, but I believe it, that it's there. I've believed since I was a girl, and I've never stopped believing.

GIULIA CAMINITO is the award-winning author of five novels. Her first novel, *The Big A*, won the Bagutta Opera Prima Prize, the Berto Prize, and the Brancati Giovani Prize. *The Bitter Water of the Lake* won the 2021 Campiello Prize and was a finalist for the Strega Prize, and has been translated into twenty-six languages worldwide. In 2024, Caminito published her most recent novel, *The Pain That Wasn't There*, which has been translated into thirteen languages. She lives in Rome.

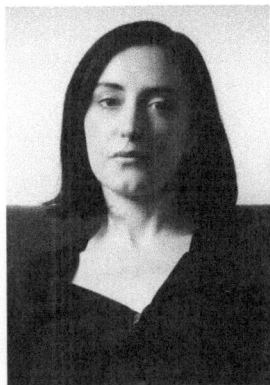

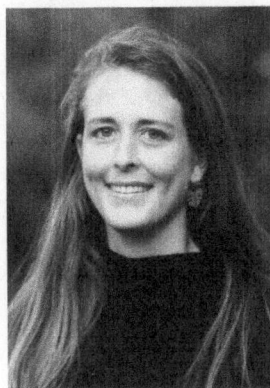

HOPE CAMPBELL GUSTAFSON's previous book-length translations include *Commander of the River* by Ubah Cristina Ali Farah and *Islands–New Islands: A Vagabond Guide to Rome* by Marco Lodoli. From Minneapolis, now living in Brooklyn, she also works for the Civitella Ranieri Foundation.

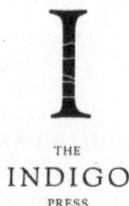

I

THE

INDIGO

PRESS

The Indigo Press is an independent publisher of contemporary
fiction and non-fiction, based in London. Guided by a spirit
of internationalism, feminism and social justice, we publish
books to make readers see the world afresh, question their
behaviour and beliefs, and imagine a better future.

Browse our books and sign up to our newsletter
for special offers and discounts:

theindigopress.com

Follow *The Indigo Press* on social media for the
latest news, events and more:

⊗ @PressIndigoThe
◎ @TheIndigoPress
ⓕ @TheIndigoPress
◉ The Indigo Press
♪ @theindigopress